Artificial Intelligence and Cloud Computing Applications in Biomedical Engineering

Biomedical engineering is undergoing a transformation because of AI, which is allowing creative solutions that enhance patient outcomes, diagnosis, treatment planning, and healthcare delivery. *Artificial Intelligence and Cloud Computing Applications in Biomedical Engineering* examines the salient characteristics of AI in biomedical engineering, highlighting its practical applications and new directions. Highlights of the book include:

- Genome sequence and visualization
- The role of AI and cloud in the detection of diseases
- Nature-inspired algorithms for disease detection
- Frameworks for disease classification

With a focus on designing AI techniques for disease detection, the book explores the role of AI in biomedical engineering. It discusses how machine learning (ML) and deep learning (DL) are at the heart of AI applications in biomedical engineering. ML algorithms, particularly those based on neural networks, enable computers to learn from large datasets, identify patterns, and make predictions or decisions without explicit programming, and implementing ML algorithms is a focus of the book. Another focus is on DL, a subset of ML, and how it uses multi-layered neural networks to achieve high accuracy in such complex tasks as image and speech recognition. Biomedical engineering generates massive amounts of data from medical imaging, genomic sequencing, wearable devices, electronic health records (EHR), and other sources. This book also discusses AI-driven big data analytics, which allows researchers and clinicians to derive meaningful insights from data, aiding in early disease detection, personalized treatment plans, and patient monitoring.

Artificial Intelligence and Cloud Computing Applications in Biomedical Engineering

Edited by H S Madhusudhan, Punit Gupta,
Pradeep Singh Rawat, and Dinesh Kumar Saini

CRC Press
Taylor & Francis Group
Boca Raton London New York

CRC Press is an imprint of the
Taylor & Francis Group, an **informa** business
AN AUERBACH BOOK

Designed cover image: Shutterstock

First edition published 2026
by CRC Press
2385 NW Executive Center Drive, Suite 320, Boca Raton FL 33431

and by CRC Press
4 Park Square, Milton Park, Abingdon, Oxon, OX14 4RN

CRC Press is an imprint of Taylor & Francis Group, LLC

ISBN: 978-1-041-01526-0 (hbk)
ISBN: 978-1-041-01926-8 (pbk)
ISBN: 978-1-003-61701-3 (ebk)

DOI: 10.1201/9781003617013

Typeset in Adobe Garamond Pro
by SPi Technologies India Pvt Ltd (Straive)

Contents

Editor Biographies

Dr. Madhusudhan H S is currently working as Associate Professor in the Department of Computer Science and Engineering at Vidyavardhaka College of Engineering, Mysuru, Karnataka, India. He has published scientific research in reputed international journals and conferences, including SCI- and Scopus-indexed journals. His areas of interest includes cloud computing, artificial intelligence, machine learning, and computer networks. He holds a doctoral degree from Visvesvaraya Technological University (VTU), Belagavi, Karnataka, India.

Dr. Punit Gupta is currently working as Assistant Professor in the Department of Computer Science and Engineering at Pandit Deendayal Energy University. He completed his post-doctoral research at University College Dublin, Ireland, and completed his PhD in Computer Science and Engineering at Jaypee University of Information Technology, Solan, India, where he is also Gold Medalist in MTech. He has research experience in internet-of-things, cloud computing, and distributed algorithms and has authored more than 80 research papers, 50+ articles and book chapters, including in peer-reviewed journals and conferences of international repute. He is a guest editor in *Recent Patent in Computer Science* journal and editorial manager of *Computer Standards & Interfaces* and the *Journal of Network and Computer Applications*. He is currently serving as a member of the Computer Society of India (CSI), a member of IEEE, and a professional member of ACM. He organized a special session on Fault-tolerant and Reliable computing in Cloud, ICIIP 2019, India, and has enthusiastically participated in and acted as an organizing committee member of numerous IEEE and other conferences.

Dr. Pradeep Singh Rawat joined the Department of Computer Science and Engineering as an assistant professor on 7 January 2010. He completed his PhD work in Computer Science and Engineering at Uttarakhand Technical University, Dehradun, India, in the year 2021, and received his MTech in Information Security and Management from the same institution, where he was also Bronze medallist in his post-graduation. He received his BTech in Computer Science and Engineering from Kumaun University, Nainital. He received the Research Excellence Award 2020–21 as well as the Outstanding Teaching award in the academic year 2022–23 on behalf of the School of Computing, at DITU. Dr. Rawat's interests center on cloud computing and its application, data communication and networking, data science applications in cloud, and soft computing. He has published and presented several research papers in various international journals and conferences of repute, including seven papers in SCIE-indexed journals with the highest impact factor (8.7), and he is an active member of the Universal Association of Computer and Electronics Engineers. He has published eight Scopus-indexed book chapters, working as an Editor with Taylor & Francis.

Prof. (Dr.) Dinesh Kumar Saini holds a PhD in Computer Science, ME in Software Systems, and MSc in Technology from one of the premier universities in India, BITS PILANI, Rajasthan, India, and is a full professor in the Department of Computer and Communication Engineering, School of Computing and Information Technology, Manipal University Jaipur, India. Dr. Saini has vast experience in academia—as a professor, researcher, and administrator—in Indian universities such as BITS Pilani and abroad, and a proven record of accomplishment of leadership skills in higher education and tertiary education sector. He served as Dean of the Faculty of Computing and Information Technology of Sohar University in the Sultanate of Oman, where he was an associate professor from 2008, and was an Adjunct Associate and Research Fellow at the University of Queensland, Brisbane Australia between 2010 and 2015. He was also the founder Program Coordinator and Head of the Department for Business Information Technology for more than 10 years. He won the Emerald Literati Award for 2018 for the article "Modeling human factors influencing herding during evacuation", published in the *International Journal of Pervasive Computing and Communications*. Besides his academic credentials aptly measured by different quantifiable metrics (e.g., Research gate score 36.36, Google citation count 976, H-Index-13, and i10 Index 22), Dr. Dinesh believes in the spirit of teamwork, thus he has consistently augmented and consolidated research capacity building at the faculty by encouraging and supporting his fellow colleagues and junior faculty members to publish in journals and conference participation that is evident in several publications that have been done in collaboration with his teammates in the faculty. He has visited the US, the UK, France, Germany, Austria, the UAE, Australia, Russia, Bahrain, and KSA for academic purposes and learned plenty of good practices in the universities of these developed countries.

Contributors

Navdeep Bhatnagar
Energy and Transportation Cluster,
    School of Business
University of Petroleum and
    Energy Studies
Dehradun, India

Amita Bisht
Department of CSE, Uttaranchal
    Institute of Technology
Uttaranchal University
Dehradun, India

Manasa C
Department of Chemistry
Vidyavardhaka College of
    Engineering
Mysuru, Karnataka, India

Divya C D
Department of Computer Science and
    Engineering
Vidyavardhaka College of Engineering
Mysuru, Karnataka, India

Abhilasha Chauhan
Department of CSE, School of
    Computing
DIT University
Dehradun, India

Kavitha D N
Department of Computer Science and
    Engineering
Vidyavardhaka College of Engineering
Mysuru, Karnataka, India

Diksha Dhiman
Department of MCA
New Horizon College of Engineering
Bengaluru, India

Pooja Gupta
School of Computing
DIT University
Dehradun, India

Chethana H T
Department of Computer Science and
    Engineering
Vidyavardhaka College of Engineering
Mysuru, Karnataka, India

Tripti Halder
Faculty of Pharmacy
DIT University
Dehradun, India

Suchi Johari
DIT University
Dehradun, Uttarakhand India

Harshitha K
Department of Computer Science and
    Engineering
Vidyavardhaka College of
    Engineering
Mysuru, Karnataka, India

Gayana J Kumar
Department of Computer Science and
    Engineering
Vidyavardhaka College of
    Engineering
Mysuru, Karnataka, India

Natesh M
Department of Computer Science and
    Engineering
Vidyavardhaka College of Engineering
Mysuru, Karnataka, India

Hamsaveni. M
Department of Computer Science and
    Engineering
Vidyavardhaka College of Engineering
Mysuru, Karnataka, India

Srabanti Maji
School of Computing
DIT University
Dehradun, India

Nishant Mathur
The Institute of Chartered Financial
    Analysts of India University
Dehradun Uttarakhand, India

Vedavathi N
Department of Computer Science and
    Engineering
Vidyavardhaka College of Engineering
Mysuru, Karnataka, India

Pradeep Singh Rawat
School of Computing
DIT University
Dehradun, India

Manju Sadasivan
School of Science and Computer Studies
CMR University
Bengaluru, India

Prateek Kumar Soni
Jaypee Institute of Information
    Technology
Noida, India

M T Vasumathi
Department of MCA
New Horizon College of Engineering
Bengaluru, India

Preface

The chapters proposed for the book include genome sequence and visualization, the role of AI and cloud in the detection of several diseases, nature-inspired algorithms for disease detection, and frameworks employed for disease classification.

The book chapter majorly focuses on

- Designing AI techniques for several disease detection.
- Exploring the role of AI in biomedical engineering.
- Implementing machine learning (ML) algorithms and models to genome detection.
- Analysis of genome sequence.

Chapter 1 emphasizes how AI helps in drug development and comprehension. AI has great potential in many areas of healthcare, particularly in research and medication creation. Large datasets may be analyzed and transformed into useful insights thanks to the incorporation of AI. By identifying novel therapeutic targets and enhancing current treatment approaches, this skill expands the field of drug discovery. Prominent pharmaceutical firms have begun integrating AI technology into their research procedures in an effort to improve their capacity to create novel medications through the use of ML and computational biology.

Chapter 2 covers various approaches is imagery from classical to advanced AI/ML and how image analysis can enhance feature extraction, genomic sequence visualization, and gene expression analysis Through practical case studies, the book shows how these techniques apply to a variety of plant genomics issues, such as transcriptome visualization, metagenomics analysis, and crop improvement, providing insights to their potential and guiding readers to develop customized solutions for specific research needs

Chapter 3 explores computational workflows, automation of bioinformatics pipelines, and integration with cloud services, supported by real-world examples that demonstrate enhanced efficiency and productivity. ML and AI's transformative impact on structural bioinformatics are examined, highlighting applications, cloud-based AI services, and future trends in predictive modeling and personalized medicine.

Chapter 4 highlights the diverse AI methodologies utilized, such as natural language processing (NLP) for symptom analysis, ML for predictive modeling, and deep learning (DL) for imaging. The results demonstrate that AI can substantially enhance the capabilities of current medical practices, paving the way for more proactive and personalized healthcare solutions. This research aims to provide a comprehensive overview of AI integration in disease management and its potential to transform the future of healthcare.

Chapter 5 covers the role of AI in medicine for the detection and prevention of various diseases. AI is revolutionizing disease detection and prevention through newer approaches like ML and DL. By analyzing diverse medical data providers such as ultrasound, MRI, mammography, genomics, and CT scans, AI enables highly accurate and rapid diagnoses, often surpassing traditional methods. AI identifies early signs of diseases like cancer, Alzheimer's, and cardiovascular conditions, providing personalized treatments based on genetic profiles, lifestyle factors, and environmental influences. AI's predictive analytics forecast disease outbreaks and individual patient risks, allowing proactive healthcare measures.

Chapter 6 aims to examine several approaches and strategies for early lung cancer detection, classification, and classification. Lung cancer often appears without symptoms in its early stages, making detection difficult. Consequently, the timely identification of cancer is crucial for improving patient outcomes. Early detection significantly enhances the likelihood of successful treatment and recovery for individuals affected by the disease.

Chapter 7 focuses on methodologies/frameworks for detecting Diabetic Retinopathy, particularly the early diagnosis and staging of DR (normal, mild, moderate, and severe), and reviews a few of the existing retinal fundus datasets. This chapter discusses the potential research gaps in DR detection/classification, highlighting areas needing further study and analysis.

Chapter 8 covers a comparative analysis of numerous state-of-the-art approaches for medical imaging diagnosis and evaluates various key qualities. The process involves assessing several critical elements, including semantic data, interpretability, visualization, and the measurement of logical linkages in medical data. Thus, we can conclude that the potential for imaging in the future will have a high degree of diagnostic accuracy for the diagnosis of various diseases, which is important for the disease's diagnosis and has a higher chance of being realized in the field of clinical diagnosis. Lastly, the applications and potential were also covered.

Chapter 9 discusses the application of advanced technology in biomedical engineering, including the conceptualization, development, and deployment of biomedical solutions. This work focuses on ML algorithms in advancements of biomedical engineering and identification and exploration of the bio fabrication, biomechanics, and biomaterials applications. The opportunities, challenges, and future enhancements in the ML algorithms for biomedical engineering are discussed in this chapter.

Chapter 10 explores the role of AI in drug discovery and development and its application in emergency and critical care through decision support systems. Robotic and automated systems, including surgical robots and AI-assisted surgeries, as well as automation in laboratory diagnostics and rehabilitation, are also discussed.

Chapter 11 presents a design to aid the blind person using edge detection. The technique aims to give the patient information about the free space apart from the obstacles around him in all directions for better mobility. The technique comprises three modules: the histogram equalization module, the segmentation module, and the Kalman filtering module. In the histogram equalization module, canny edge detector is employed to detect edges and subsequently, histogram equalization is carried out. Furthermore, adaptive region growth is employed in the segmentation module to complete the segmentation process.

We hope that the works published in this book will be able to serve the concerned communities of ML and healthcare society.

Acknowledgment

The editors are thankful to the authors and reviewers of the concerned chapters who contributed to this book with their scientific work and useful comments, respectively.

Chapter 1

Artificial Intelligence and Computational Biology in Drug Discovery

Manasa C, Madhusudhan H S and Punit Gupta

1.1 Introduction

The average small-molecule medicine takes around 15 years and almost $2 billion to produce before it reaches the market, demonstrating the high level of research and financial investment required for traditional drug design [1]. The complicated nature of biologics, target validation, and hit identification procedures are to blame for this drawn-out process and high expense. By increasing efficacy, efficiency, and accuracy, recent developments in computational approaches—such as computational biology, computer-aided drug design (CADD), and artificial intelligence (AI)—are transforming drug discovery and increasing the number of new drugs that are approved for sale.

The pharmaceutical industry is rapidly changing due to AI, especially in the area of medication discovery. AI technologies can increase the efficacy and efficiency of pharmaceutical research by utilizing aggregated data. This study emphasizes how AI helps in drug development and comprehension. AI has great potential in many areas of healthcare, particularly in research and medication creation. Large datasets may be analyzed and transformed into useful insights thanks to the incorporation of AI. By identifying novel therapeutic targets and enhancing current treatment approaches, this skill expands the field of drug discovery. Prominent pharmaceutical firms have begun integrating AI technology into their research procedures in an effort to improve their capacity to create novel medications through the use of machine learning (ML) and computational biology. This greatly cuts down on the time and expense required to introduce novel treatments to the market. The objective of applying AI to medication research is to forecast a compound's molecular activity and evaluate its possible safety and efficacy. AI systems can find viable medication candidates more quickly by evaluating genomic data, clinical trials, and electronic health records. This reduces the need for needless testing. Because pharmaceutical researchers have access to large datasets from multiple sources that may be efficiently evaluated by sophisticated AI systems, data usage is essential in drug development. AI can gain new insights and improve the drug discovery process because of this abundance of data, which includes high-resolution medical pictures and clinical trials. To improve medication development, AI technologies are being combined more and more with insights from pharmacology and structural biology. AI's potential for finding novel treatments can be fully achieved by utilizing insights from a variety of scientific fields, which holds promise for major improvements in patient care and treatment results. With its ability to enhance pharmacological data analysis and expedite procedures, AI has become a crucial component of contemporary drug discovery initiatives. AI improves both ligand-based and structure-based virtual screening (VS) processes, improving scoring functions and broadening the search field for new compounds, especially when applied to ML and deep learning models [2]. Nowadays, during the discovery stage, computational techniques are essential for locating possible therapeutic targets and refining lead compounds. By evaluating enormous volumes of biological data, computational approaches have the advantage of speeding up the research and development process and potentially identifying novel therapeutic possibilities. These techniques lower drug development costs and raise the possibility of finding promising therapeutic candidates, including molecular modeling and in silico ADMET predictions [3]. The use of computer methods in drug design is fraught with difficulties, though, including the requirement for reliable data, the possibility of inaccurate predictive modeling, and the difficulty of combining different computational approaches. Ensuring the precision and speed of computational screenings becomes crucial as chemical libraries grow in size and diversity. Drug development has been transformed by the advent of computer methods such as ML and molecular dynamics (MD) simulations. By modeling and analyzing interactions at the molecular level, MD simulations give researchers insights into the thermodynamics and kinetics of protein-ligand binding. Through the prediction of binding affinities and the validation of computational docking studies, these techniques improve lead compound development. To expedite the drug discovery process, CADD makes use of a variety of computational techniques. Finding and improving lead compounds from sizable chemical databases is a major function of VS, which emphasizes both structure-based and ligand-based approaches. Scientists can swiftly refine candidate profiles thanks to this method, which also speeds up the process of finding new medication candidates and repurposing existing ones.

The phases of drug discovery, clinical testing, and regulatory approval are all part of the intricate and multifaceted process of drug research and development. The accuracy, efficacy, and efficiency of this process have greatly increased with the integration of AI and computational techniques, especially when it comes to finding novel medications and customizing patient care. Less than 15% of medications advance through clinical trials successfully, despite substantial resources being devoted to drug discovery [4]. In about half of cases, failures are primarily caused by poor pharmacokinetic characteristics, such as toxicity and absorption [5]. Therefore, a key area of further research and development is effectively identifying promising therapeutic candidates. The integration of cutting-edge computational techniques and AI technology, which has enormous potential to speed up the discovery and development of new treatments, is where precision medicine is headed. The future of personalized medicine in the treatment of cancer is expected to be greatly influenced by this continuous innovation, which is essential in tackling the difficulties encountered in drug development. In order to improve patient outcomes in the healthcare industry and expedite pharmaceutical development, more investigation and integration of these technologies are necessary.

1.2 Computational Biology in Drug Design

Modern drug design heavily relies on computational biology, especially in the early phases of drug discovery. Researchers can learn a great deal about the causes of diseases and the impacts of possible treatment candidates by combining several interdisciplinary approaches and computational techniques. In order to comprehend pathogenic pathways and overcome medication resistance, methods like density functional theory (DFT), quantum mechanics (QM), and MD simulations are essential. Finding possible biological targets is the first step in modern drug development, and this process frequently involves a number of scientific fields, such as structural biology, molecular biology, cell biology, genomics, proteomics, computational biology, and bioinformatics. Because it sheds light on how disease arises and advances, an understanding of pathogenesis is essential for both drug discovery and treatment development. By deciphering the cellular and molecular processes behind illness, scientists can increase the precision of their drug development initiatives.

MD simulations, QM, and molecular mechanics (MM) are examples of computational chemistry techniques that are frequently used in medicinal chemistry and computational biology. By enabling energy calculations and molecular interaction simulations, these techniques enable a more thorough investigation of biological systems and help define how medications interact with their targets [6]. MD simulations are effective for examining pathogenic pathways and tackling drug resistance issues, in conjunction with DFT and QM techniques [7]. They give scientists the ability to model the actual motions of atoms and molecules, which help them understand how proteins and other biomolecules behave dynamically in real-time settings. Studying pathogenic pathways, using molecular docking to anticipate how medications will bind to their targets, and improving lead compounds to increase their efficacy are important areas of attention in drug discovery. Computational technologies speed up drug discovery and increase the likelihood of successful clinical applications by simplifying these procedures.

1.2.1 Application of MM in Drug Design

A key strategy in drug design is MM, which uses classical mechanics to examine molecule interactions while preserving the computer power frequently needed for quantum mechanical computations. By supporting target identification, molecular docking, lead optimization, and the use of coarse-grained (CG) models, this method has greatly improved our understanding of ligand-protein dynamics. Researchers can learn more about the molecular mechanisms underpinning drug efficacy, resistance, and interactions by integrating MM with MD simulations. This knowledge will ultimately help guide the development of more effective therapeutic treatments. MD simulations, which use algorithms like Verlet's Algorithm and Leap-frog Algorithm to model the paths of biomacromolecules in a solvent environment, are very important in drug discovery [8]. When assessing ligand–protein interactions, MD can provide time-dependent characteristics and aid in visualizing the dynamic behavior of proteins. In order to adequately depict the system prior to simulation, the initial protein structure is usually determined by experimental techniques like cryo-electron microscopy (Cryo-EM) or X-ray crystallography [9].

Compounds are positioned into certain binding sites via molecular docking based on energy interactions and spatial complementarity. By drastically cutting down on the time and expenses involved in finding possible hits, VS improves the drug discovery process. The precision of docking poses and binding affinity evaluations, which are aided by MD simulations that take target protein and ligand flexibility into account, are crucial to the success of VS [10].

Optimizing therapeutic candidates requires precise modeling of ligand–target interactions. MD simulations provide an in-depth understanding of these interactions, aiding in the identification of crucial binding residues and enabling changes to improve medication efficacy. The optimization of AKT inhibitors and bedaquiline are noteworthy examples that highlight MD's function in improving binding affinities and minimizing side effects [11]. CG models are especially helpful for examining intricate biomolecular processes like oligomerization and membrane interactions because they offer a straightforward yet efficient way to investigate long-duration and large-scale processes in molecular systems [12]. A common CG technique in drug design is the Martini force field, which lowers processing requirements and improves the effectiveness of molecular mechanism exploration [13].

By combining MM and MD simulations, the drug discovery process can be greatly accelerated, resulting in more effective pharmacological intervention identification and development.

1.2.2 Application of QM in Drug Design

A vital technique in drug design, QM offers an electronic-level investigation of therapeutic targets that improves comprehension and optimization procedures. Researchers can more precisely anticipate binding modes, enhance scoring functions, and eventually create more potent medicinal medicines by combining QM with MM and MD simulations. Even with its high computing cost, QM has a lot of potential to solve problems with conventional drug design techniques, especially when dealing with intricate biomolecular systems [14]. Detailed knowledge about possible drug targets is crucial for lead discovery and optimization, as well as for later stages of drug design, according to structural studies. Effective binding mode prediction is frequently achieved through the use of molecular docking and pharmacophore models, which enable speedy evaluation of possible ligand–target interactions and speedier discovery of promising therapeutic options. A technique for flexible and logical docking that thoroughly examines ligand–target interactions is MD simulations. However, MD simulations still have limits, particularly when it comes to enzymes or drug targets that contain metals where valence electron transfer takes place. This disparity calls into question the validity of conventional approaches in these intricate situations.

These issues can be resolved by using QM, which makes it possible to examine pharmacological targets at the electronic level. Its use in metal-containing proteins and enzyme research is growing in popularity, demonstrating its capacity to elucidate molecular pathways important to drug design [15]. Novel drug designs, such as the creation of high-affinity ligands for FKBP12 and inhibitors for human DHFR, have benefited greatly from the use of QM techniques [16]. QM techniques, including semiempirical QM scoring functions and QM-polarized ligand docking, have been integrated into improved scoring systems in drug design.

Although QM calculations provide accurate information, their processing demands restrict their applicability to smaller systems, usually consisting of a few hundred atoms. To get beyond these restrictions, more development in quantum computing approaches to drug creation is required.

1.3 Computer-Aided Drug Design

More than 70 authorized medications have been discovered thanks to CADD, which uses two main approaches: ligand-based drug design (LBDD) and structure-based drug design (SBDD). By using a target molecule's three-dimensional (3D) structure to investigate ligand–target interactions, SBDD helps researchers create and improve medications by taking into account the target's unique geometry and active sites, which improves the precision of drug binding predictions. In contrast, LBDD is used in situations where the target's three-dimensional structure is unavailable. It begins with a known molecule or group of known effective molecules and uses knowledge of the structural-activity relationship (SAR) to optimize and find possible drug candidates. In lead discovery, SBDD and LBDD are both crucial approaches that serve different purposes in the drug design process. The technique used for drug candidate development is influenced by the availability of structural information about the target, which is a major factor in the decision between them. More than 70 authorized medications have been developed, thanks in large part to CADD, which represents a major breakthrough in pharmacology and drug development [17]. The approval history of medications, which begins with Captopril in 1981 and continues to more recent medications like Remdesivir in 2021, demonstrates the ongoing importance of CADD in therapeutic innovation [18].

1.3.1 Structure-Based Drug Design

One method for identifying and optimizing leads in drug discovery is called Structure-Based Drug Design (SBDD). It uses methods including structure-based VS, molecular docking, and MD simulations to analyze ligand–target interactions and binding affinities. By using methodical techniques such as target preparation, binding site identification, compound library preparation, molecular docking, and scoring, SBDD has helped find a number of authorized medications. Target protein structures are now more readily available in the Protein Data Bank (PDB) as a result of developments in structural biology. To anticipate target structures based on amino acid sequences, computational techniques like homology modeling, AlphaFold, and ab initio protein structure prediction have been developed [19]. When a template is not available, ab initio techniques use primary sequences to save energy and optimize structures [20].

Effective molecular docking, which can be achieved by methods like site-directed mutagenesis and co-crystallized complex analysis, requires the discovery of binding sites. When current information on binding sites is lacking, blind docking techniques are utilized, which necessitate a thorough sample of the protein surface in order to anticipate possible binding modes. In order to guarantee oral bioactivity and advantageous drug-like qualities, compounds from different libraries are filtered using Veber criteria and Lipinski's "Rule of Five" [21]. Compound libraries are essential for VS. Alongside VS, molecular docking and scoring are widely used to expedite the search for promising drug candidates. This procedure is facilitated by tools like AutoDock, GLIDE, and DOCK6, with various docking strategies based on the ligand and target structures' degree of flexibility. When compared to more conventional methods, more recent techniques that use deep learning, like EquiBind and DiffDock, improve speed and accuracy in binding mode prediction [22]. In

SBDD, MD simulations are essential because they improve target protein flexibility and provide precise binding affinity assessments. They aid in the improvement of compound ranking in lead optimization initiatives and offer insights into ligand–target interactions. When used in conjunction with free energy estimates, MD simulations can be especially useful for thoroughly assessing binding affinities. The incorporation of these approaches into SBDD highlights its importance in contemporary drug discovery and development, expediting procedures and encouraging therapeutic innovation.

1.3.2 Ligand-Based Drug Design

When target structures are not available, LBDD is a useful strategy in drug discovery. This approach finds structural and physicochemical characteristics linked to biological activity by using known active chemicals against certain targets. Pharmacophore modeling and Quantitative Structure–Activity Relationship (QSAR) analysis are important LBDD approaches that help with the creation and optimization of novel drugs. In order to understand interactions with particular targets, pharmacophore modeling derives chemical characteristics from known bioactive conformations of ligands. Catalyst, LigandScout, and MOE are notable pharmacophore modeling tools that help identify ligands with comparable interactions but distinct scaffolds. However, because they are static and reduce complicated interactions to geometric aspects, conventional pharmacophore models have drawbacks. The dynophore technique, which combines MD simulations and pharmacophore modeling to overcome these obstacles, provides a more sophisticated depiction of ligand binding by investigating different binding modes and their frequencies throughout simulations. Based on the idea that biological activity is intrinsically connected to structural characteristics, QSAR analysis investigates the relationship between ligand bioactivities and these characteristics. To provide accurate predictions, a robust QSAR model needs a sufficient dataset, appropriate training and testing compound selection, avoidance of autocorrelated descriptors, and validation. According to the dimensionality of the descriptors, QSAR techniques can be categorized as follows: 1D-QSAR links bioactivity to global chemical properties; 2D-QSAR concentrates on structural features without taking 3D into account and then moves from 3D to 6D-QSAR that includes more intricate depictions of ligand conformations and interactions. Regression analysis and artificial neural networks (ANNs) are two methods used in QSAR approaches, which can be either linear or nonlinear and build predictive models. Notwithstanding its benefits, QSAR has drawbacks, namely with regard to the descriptor constraints and the availability of high-quality datasets required for trustworthy model creation. Ongoing studies aim to improve the extraction of significant structural characterizations in drug design by integrating new descriptors and approaches. The effective design and optimization of novel medicinal compounds are greatly aided by LBDD, especially through pharmacophore modeling and QSAR, thanks to these methods and ongoing developments.

1.4 Applications of Artificial Intelligence in the Identification of Drugs

Through improvements in VS techniques, AI has had a major impact on drug identification. By using ML techniques to optimize ligand–receptor interactions, these methods improve the efficacy, precision, and predictive power of drug discovery procedures. Finding promising drug candidates and reducing incorrect predictions depend heavily on AI-driven advancements in scoring features and interaction with current VS methods. The purpose of the VS pipeline is to increase the efficiency and predictability of discovering possible small molecules while lowering the cost of high-throughput screening. In order to streamline drug identification procedures, this pipeline makes use of ML and AI techniques that enable a robust generalization process over several VS phases. The two categories of VS are structure-based and ligand-based VS. While structure-based methods function without the use of structural information from ligand-receptor binding, ligand-based VS makes use of it. AI's potential to advance both forms of VS is highlighted by the breadth of its applications in this field. Advanced AI algorithms based on nonparametric scoring functions have been used to generate improvements in structure-based VS techniques. These techniques use available experimental data to find correlations between feature vectors and protein-ligand binding free energy. Researchers can identify significant nonlinear interactions and create scoring functions with good generalization capabilities thanks to this data-driven methodology.

Numerous AI-based scoring functions, such as ANN-based NNScore, SVM-based ID-score, and RF-based RF-score, have surfaced. These scoring algorithms surpass traditional methods in binding affinity predictions and show excellent accuracy in identifying putative ligands [23]. Leading AI techniques use a number of important algorithms, including feed-forward ANNs, random forests (RF), Bayesian approaches, support vector machines (SVM), and deep neural networks, to enhance scoring function performance [24]. Strong RF-based prediction software was developed as a result of research by Ballester et al. that concentrated on improving AI-based non-predetermined scoring functions to provide higher binding affinity predictions for protein-ligand complexes [25]. Another noteworthy advancement in this field is the PROFILER automated procedure, which finds high-probability binding sites for bioactive substances. AI's ability to score tasks in structure-based VS has demonstrated a high level of effectiveness in locating targets. Characterizing the physicochemical characteristics and structural features of target proteins to improve candidate selection and predicting accuracy, as well as improving the post-processing of scoring computations using ML models, are future directions in AI-Enhanced VS.

1.5 Enhanced Molecular Dynamics Simulations with Artificial Intelligence

One important development in computational chemistry is the combination of AI and MD simulations. This collaboration improves atomic-scale simulations' accuracy and efficiency while offering deep insights into molecular interactions and biological activities. Researchers are well-positioned to use the latest advancements in AI algorithms and computational methods to overcome long-standing obstacles in complex system modeling and expedite drug discovery procedures. One essential tool for examining the structure and biochemical characteristics of diverse systems is computational chemistry. The ability to monitor atomic-level movements in biomolecular systems through the use of techniques like MD simulations has proven crucial for comprehending molecular behavior in a variety of settings. However, because of the processing power needed for such simulations, it is still difficult to analyze the movement of large groups of atoms. Conventional methods are limited in their ability to analyze complex molecular systems over long periods of time due to their high computing resource requirements. By improving simulation capabilities, the incorporation of AI technology into computational chemistry seeks to address these computational issues. AI has the ability to perform large volumes of simulations more successfully than conventional techniques because it can process and evaluate the enormous volumes of data produced by simulations in an efficient manner. The investigation of intricate molecular interactions is made easier by this integration, which enables notable increases in simulation speed and accuracy.

Building neural network potentials, especially with Behler–Parrinello symmetry functions, is a prominent use of AI in this field. Due to their ability to evaluate thousands of atoms at once, these models are extremely useful for researching high-dimensional systems and offering crucial insights into the behavior of molecules [26]. Recent research has shown how well AI-enhanced MD can solve a number of challenging scientific issues, such as complex Schrödinger equation solvation analyses, machine-learned density functional development, and chemical trajectory data classification. Additionally, AI methods have been used to forecast molecular characteristics, especially when evaluating excited state electrons and developing many-body theories.

1.6 De Novo Drug Design by AI

One important advancement in drug discovery procedures is de novo drug design, which is fueled by AI. This strategy seeks to overcome conventional limits in drug design techniques by producing novel compounds with desired chemical properties through the use of sophisticated ML frameworks. Advanced data processing, generative modeling, and optimization are some of the methods used, with the ultimate goal of bridging the gap between intricate molecular interactions and potent therapeutic medicines. A thorough method that includes several stages, including target identification, binding site prediction, and molecular docking, is demonstrated by the incorporation of ML into de novo drug creation. To precisely anticipate ligand binding positions and orientations, algorithms such as EquiBind and DiffDock use diffusion generative approaches and geometric deep learning techniques [27]. AI successfully addresses the difficulties of finding and creating new medication candidates, despite the complexity and size of the chemical universe. Data selection from publicly accessible databases is the first step in the ML architecture used in drug creation. Next, properties are filtered, and molecules with the necessary attributes are isolated by classification. Molecular structures and attributes are encoded using methods such as graphical representations and the Simplified Molecular Input Line Entry System (SMILES). To improve molecular generation processes, sophisticated generative models are optimized through the use of property prediction techniques and reinforcement learning. Recent developments that use AI to learn the distribution of molecular data have fueled generative techniques in drug creation. This generative method works especially well for ligand- and structure-oriented generation. Effective molecular design is made possible by the capacity to customize molecules based on complex structural interactions with target proteins, which highlights the significance of thorough structural data during model training. Using comprehensive structural data about the ligands and proteins, structure-oriented generation focuses on creating new compounds that bind to particular proteins efficiently. Iterative changes to initial scaffolds are made in approaches like fragment-based techniques in order to maximize binding interactions and therapeutic efficacy. Notable models that use this method are G-SchNet and DeepLigBuilder, which use 3D structures to enable precise molecule production [28]. The goal of ligand-oriented generation is to create novel compounds with ideal characteristics while guaranteeing a high binding affinity for certain target proteins. Using strategies like autoencoders and reinforcement learning, this technology optimizes a number of molecular parameters, including ADMET, synthetic accessibility, and clearance, while enabling the exploration of latent chemical regions through known active compounds.

In AI-based drug creation, datasets and descriptors are essential for building trustworthy generative models. Effective ML model training requires knowledge about molecular structures, characteristics, and biological information, all of which can be found in high-quality molecular data from databases such as ChEMBL, PubChem, and DrugBank. For molecule generation, deep learning methods—specifically, Generative Adversarial Networks (GANs) and Variational Autoencoders (VAEs)—are widely used. A crucial stage in the drug design process is property optimization, which uses ML approaches to improve qualities like solubility and drug-likeness. Effective optimization based on predictive models is made possible by techniques like reinforcement learning, which raise the possibility that produced compounds will satisfy therapeutic requirements. In de novo drug design, thorough evaluation metrics are essential for determining the caliber of synthesized compounds. AI-driven medication design makes a significant contribution to the pharmaceutical industry because of this methodical evaluation and strict optimization.

1.7 Statistics on Drug Discovery and AI Usage

The figures help stakeholders make well-informed decisions about research, development, and investment by offering a framework for comprehending the expanding importance of AI in revolutionizing drug discovery and the larger pharmaceutical landscape. Important data on drug discovery, with an emphasis on the function of AI in the pharmaceutical sector, may be found in Table 1.1 [29]. It contains information on the market sizes for AI applications in the pharmaceutical sector, the success rates of drug development throughout various stages, and how AI technologies are improving drug discovery procedures. The percentage of medications that make it through clinical trials from start to finish is known as the success rate. The overall success rate of traditional drug development is only about 10–15%, which means that only a tiny percentage of substances investigated will finally make it to market. AI is working to raise these rates by increasing the effectiveness of finding interesting candidates and expediting certain stages of the drug development process. The financial environment around the use of AI in drug

Table 1.1   Significant statistics related to success rates, market sizes, and the impact of AI on drug discovery processes

Statistic	Value/Details
Success Rate (Phase I to II)	52%
AI-Discovered Drugs Phase 1 Success Rate	80–90%, significantly higher than historical averages of 40–65%
Overall Clinical Drug Development Success Rate	10–15%
Global AI in Drug Discovery Market Size	USD 1.5 billion in 2023, anticipated to grow at a CAGR of 29.7% from 2024 to 2030
Estimated Cost and Time Savings through AI	25–50% reduction in time and cost
Number of AI-Applicated Investigational Drugs	164 investigational drugs and 1 approved drug
Most Common AI Use Cases	Drug molecule discovery (76%), drug target discovery (22%), clinical outcomes analysis (3%)
Expected Growth in AI Market (2022–2029)	Projected increase from $13.8 billion to $164.1 billion
AI Use in Clinical Trials	Enhanced productivity and reduction in cycle times

discovery is indicated by market sizes. According to estimations, the global market for AI in drug discovery is worth about USD 1.5 billion as of 2023, and it is expected to increase significantly over the next several years. This market data shows the pharmaceutical industry's growing investment in and acceptance of AI technology, pointing to a move toward data-driven approaches that offer better treatment results and higher returns on investment. The table shows measurable advantages, including time and cost reductions as well as qualitative enhancements in the drug discovery process.

1.8 Drug Resistance

Drug resistance is a serious problem since microorganisms develop ways to avoid the effects of medications, particularly when antimicrobial medicines are being developed. The development of new therapeutic compounds that can circumvent or overcome these resistance mechanisms has become necessary due to the proliferation of multi-drug-resistant bacteria, which has made treating illnesses more difficult. By examining genomic data from resistant strains, computational biology plays a crucial role in describing the genetic and molecular foundations of drug resistance. This allows for the creation of targeted medicines that can get around resistance mechanisms and enhance treatment results. AI improves this procedure by making it easier to analyze big datasets and forecast possible pathogen resistance patterns. By finding patterns and connections in microbial genomes, ML algorithms can forecast the likelihood that a particular bacterium would become resistant to a particular medication. Drug design and the choice of suitable treatment approaches can both be influenced by this predictive ability.

Nevertheless, AI and computational techniques have drawbacks. For example, prediction accuracy is highly dependent on the caliber and variety of data provided. Models may produce false findings if training datasets are biased or lacking, which could have a negative impact on the creation of successful treatments [30]. Computational biologists, microbiologists, and doctors must work together and use interdisciplinary approaches to effectively address drug resistance. Researchers can create more successful experimental investigations and clinical trials aimed at overcoming resistance by merging knowledge from several disciplines and utilizing AI techniques and computational models.

1.9 Complications in Drug Discovery by AI and Computational Methods

Despite its potential advantages, the integration of computational techniques and AI in drug discovery poses a number of difficulties that may impede advancement. The landscape of drug development is complicated by elements like data quality, algorithm biases, computational resource needs, the complexities of biological systems, and regulatory obstacles. It is essential to comprehend these issues in order to improve methods and boost drug development effectiveness. The main issues with drug development with AI and computational techniques are data availability and quality. Biased, inconsistent, or incomplete datasets can have a big impact on AI model results, producing poor drug candidates and inaccurate forecasts. Furthermore, depending too much on past data may unintentionally reinforce preexisting biases, distorting outcomes and impeding the development of novel treatments. Health disparities in pharmacological efficacy can be reinforced by algorithmic biases present in training data, which can result in suboptimal therapies for underrepresented populations [31]. Significant resources are needed for computational approaches, especially when working with complex biological systems and gigascale libraries. Large virtual library screening can be very expensive and time-consuming, which restricts access to cutting-edge drug discovery technologies. Computational methods face a major obstacle in biological complexity since oversimplifying models and assumptions might result in inaccurate predictions of drug activity in vivo. Finding promising therapeutic candidates might be challenging due to the unforeseen results that can arise from biological systems' dynamic nature. Regulatory obstacles may impede the development of new treatments by delaying the conversion of AI discoveries into clinical applications. There are both technological and cultural obstacles when combining AI and computational techniques with conventional methods. New computational approaches may be resisted by researchers used to traditional laboratory methods, which would prevent cooperation and knowledge exchange. In clinical trials, where almost 90% of candidates fail to receive market approval, high failure rates continue to be a major problem in drug discovery [32]. Reliance on computational techniques does not ensure success because the discovery process may still be beset by weak ligand properties and insufficient target validation. Although AI and computational approaches have enormous potential to transform drug discovery, these issues must be resolved to maximize their usefulness and boost the effectiveness of introducing novel treatments to the market.

1.10 Computational Methods and AI for Variant Classification

These methods prioritize and forecast the functional impact of different genetic changes by utilizing large biological datasets, ML algorithms, and integrative methodologies. In clinical genomics, these developments are especially important for the development of customized treatment and the detection of uncommon genetic illnesses. Classifying variants entails determining how genetic changes affect phenotypes and illnesses. Computational techniques are now crucial for classifying variations, especially those that result in uncommon genetic illnesses, because of the enormous amount of genetic data produced by high-throughput sequencing.

The accuracy and speed of categorization attempts are improved by ML, AI-driven algorithms, and conventional annotation techniques. ML models and rule-based systems are two computational methods for variant annotation. While ML techniques learn from massive datasets to find patterns and outcomes linked to particular mutations, rule-based annotation makes use of current biological knowledge to forecast the possible functional implications of variants. Prominent instances of rule-based applications in the field are tools like ANNOVAR and the Ensembl Variant Effect Predictor (VEP) [33]. Variant categorization has made substantial use of ML models, particularly supervised learning methods. These algorithms can accurately forecast the functional effects of novel variants by training on labeled datasets of known harmful and benign variants. SVM and RF are two well-liked algorithms that find distinctive characteristics that are correlated with clinical importance. When it comes to managing the intricate relationships between various genomic characteristics and how they affect variant classification, AI models are especially useful.

Improved classification accuracy has been shown with integrative approaches that use a variety of algorithms and aggregate data from several sources. To evaluate the impact of variants, techniques such as CADD make use of a larger collection of annotations, such as functional genomic data and evolutionary conservation. Improving the accuracy of variant categorization in clinical situations requires addressing these constraints. AI developments like neural networks and reinforcement learning present exciting opportunities to improve prediction models and deepen our comprehension of intricate variation effects.

1.11 Outlook

Determining precision medicines that could improve patients' general health and quality of life while they receive treatment requires an understanding of genetic pathways. Because traditional drug discovery techniques are frequently expensive and time-consuming, a more effective strategy is required. A quick way to find precise medications catered to particular genetic variations is using computational biology. The many stages of the drug discovery process are greatly impacted by the computational tools and software available today. Through an organized methodology, computational techniques aid in the identification of precision medications that are aligned with specific genetic variants. The collection of genetic variants, pathogenicity prediction, three-dimensional protein structure modeling, molecular docking with standard drugs, VS for specific drug identification, and MD simulation are all components of the combined methodology for finding precision drugs. The comprehension of pharmacological efficacy is improved by this integrated approach. However, in order to maximize the identification process for precision pharmaceuticals, it is imperative that present computational methodologies be drastically overhauled. The procedures involved in medication design and discovery could be completely transformed by AI. One prominent example is the Chapel Hill Eshelman School of Pharmacy's Reinforcement Learning for Structural Evolution (ReLeaSE) system, which uses neural networks and algorithms to teach and improve the process of finding promising drug candidates [34]. AI enhances traditional data analysis, which frequently concentrates on smaller datasets related to diseases, and helps with the logical discovery and improvement of treatments based on large datasets. This has a favorable impact on precision medicine. AI technology can help with biomarker identification, diagnostic improvement, and the development of new medications in addition to drug discovery. AI's significant impact on the future of healthcare is demonstrated by its use in the development of target-based precision medications.

1.12 Conclusion

Drug design has been greatly aided by computational biology techniques, especially in fields like lead optimization, VS, mechanism studies, and target discovery. These approaches have strong theoretical foundations, and the majority of the training data required for deep learning comes from computational biology methods. For studying thermodynamic and kinetic properties and comprehending molecular mechanisms, MD simulations—including force field-based and ab initio simulations—remain essential. MD simulations are still required to accurately assess binding energies or free energy changes for ligand–target interactions as well as to characterize the structural and dynamic characteristics of targets. Though accuracy is frequently compromised, molecular force field simulations can be scaled to bigger systems. This restriction is lessened by the QM/MM method, which is being used more and more in drug discovery. Larger-scale applications, especially for ab initio techniques, may be hampered by the high processing requirements of MD simulations. CG techniques have been developed and successfully used in a variety of scenarios to mitigate the problem of computational expenses. Drug development has been expedited with the advent and broad application of CADD, molecular docking, VS, and QSAR tools. Significant advancements have been made in the traditional paradigms of drug design with the incorporation of AI methodologies. This is especially true in molecular generation through generative models that use molecular graphs or representations like SMILES and SELFIES, which have gained popularity because of their efficacy in molecular optimization tasks. Numerous issues still exist with the AI frameworks in use today, despite improvements in computational modeling and AI techniques for drug creation. Concerns have been raised about whether models actually learn patterns from their training sets, and the assessment of molecular generators is impacted by particular compound datasets. Furthermore, many datasets are of poor quality and do not satisfy the thorough standards of actual drug research. Molecular representation is essential for efficient molecular learning and generation, as well as for improving benchmarks and assessment metrics.

Molecules are often represented as traditional two-dimensional (2D) graphs, which are ideal for processing by GNNs. Three-dimensional (3D) representations, like point clouds, 3D graphs, and 3D grids, have received more attention recently since they are essential for capturing spatial information. Now that macromolecules pose more difficulties, researchers must add more units to molecular generators to account for Euclidean symmetries—specifically rotational, translational, and reflectional symmetries—suitable for the complexity of small molecular systems. Creating pre-trained Molecular Representation Models, incorporating domain expertise, and utilizing a variety of data sources are three exciting avenues for further study in AI-driven drug creation. All things considered, the incorporation of AI and computational biology into the drug design framework presents promising opportunities, despite persistent obstacles and room for further development.

References

[1] Hemel, D. J., & Ouellette, L. L. (2023). Valuing medical innovation. *Stanford Law Review*, *75*, 517.

[2] Oliveira, T. A. D., Silva, M. P. D., Maia, E. H. B., Silva, A. M. D., & Taranto, A. G. (2023). Virtual screening algorithms in drug discovery: A review focused on machine and deep learning methods. *Drugs and Drug Candidates*, *2*(2), 311–334.

[3] Sadybekov, A. V., & Katritch, V. (2023). Computational approaches streamlining drug discovery. *Nature*, *616*(7958), 673–685.

[4] Michaeli, D. T., Michaeli, T., Albers, S., Boch, T., & Michaeli, J. C. (2024). Special FDA designations for drug development: Orphan, fast track, accelerated approval, priority review, and breakthrough therapy. *The European Journal of Health Economics*, *25*, 979–997.

[5] Morales Castro, D., Dresser, L., Granton, J., & Fan, E. (2023). Pharmacokinetic alterations associated with critical illness. *Clinical Pharmacokinetics*, *62*(2), 209–220.

[6] Peluso, P., & Chankvetadze, B. (2023). Recent developments in molecular modeling tools and applications related to pharmaceutical and biomedical research. *Journal of Pharmaceutical and Biomedical Analysis*, *238*, 115836.

[7] van der Kamp, M. W., & Begum, J. (2024). QM/MM for structure-based drug design: Techniques and applications. *Computational Drug Discovery: Methods and Applications*, *1*, 119–156.

[8] Hu, X., Zeng, Z., Zhang, J., Wu, D., Li, H., & Geng, F. (2023). Molecular dynamics simulation of the interaction of food proteins with small molecules. *Food Chemistry*, *405*, 134824.

[9] Patil, V. M., Gupta, S. P., Masand, N., & Balasubramanian, K. (2024). Experimental and computational models to understand protein-ligand, metal-ligand and metal-DNA interactions pertinent to targeted cancer and other therapies. *European Journal of Medicinal Chemistry Reports*, *10*, 100133.

[10] Gu, S., Shen, C., Yu, J., Zhao, H., Liu, H., Liu, L., ... & Kang, Y. (2023). Can molecular dynamics simulations improve predictions of protein-ligand binding affinity with machine learning?. *Briefings in Bioinformatics*, *24*(2), bbad008.

[11] Mi, J., Wu, X., & Liang, J. (2024). The advances in adjuvant therapy for tuberculosis with immunoregulatory compounds. *Frontiers in Microbiology, 15,* 1380848.

[12] Torrens-Fontanals, M., Stepniewski, T. M., Aranda-García, D., Morales-Pastor, A., Medel-Lacruz, B., & Selent, J. (2020). How do molecular dynamics data complement static structural data of GPCRs. *International Journal of Molecular Sciences, 21*(16), 5933.

[13] Stone, J. E., Phillips, J. C., Freddolino, P. L., Hardy, D. J., Trabuco, L. G., & Schulten, K. (2007). Accelerating molecular modeling applications with graphics processors. *Journal of Computational Chemistry, 28*(16), 2618–2640.

[14] Manathunga, M., Götz, A. W., & Merz Jr, K. M. (2022). Computer-aided drug design, quantum-mechanical methods for biological problems. *Current Opinion in Structural Biology, 75,* 102417.

[15] Palermo, G., Spinello, A., Saha, A., & Magistrato, A. (2021). Frontiers of metal-coordinating drug design. *Expert Opinion on Drug Discovery, 16*(5), 497–511.

[16] Reddy, M. R., & Erion, M. D. (Eds.). (2001). *Free energy calculations in rational drug design.* Springer Science & Business Media.

[17] Dar, K. B., Bhat, A. H., Amin, S., Hamid, R., Anees, S., Anjum, S., … & Ganie, S. A. (2018). Modern computational strategies for designing drugs to curb human diseases: A prospect. *Current Topics in Medicinal Chemistry, 18*(31), 2702–2719.

[18] Geronikaki, A., Dubey, G., Petrou, A., & Kirubakaran, S. (2023). Computer-aided drug design: an overview. In *Cheminformatics, QSAR and machine learning applications for novel drug development,* 39–68, Elsevier.

[19] Bertoline, L. M., Lima, A. N., Krieger, J. E., & Teixeira, S. K. (2023). Before and after AlphaFold2: An overview of protein structure prediction. *Frontiers in Bioinformatics, 3,* 1120370.

[20] Karamertzanis, P. G., & Pantelides, C. C. (2007). Ab initio crystal structure prediction. II. Flexible molecules. *Molecular Physics, 105*(2–3), 273–291.

[21] Khan, T., Ahmad, R., Azad, I., Raza, S., Joshi, S., & Khan, A. R. (2018). Computer-aided drug design and virtual screening of targeted combinatorial libraries of mixed-ligand transition metal complexes of 2-butanone thiosemicarbazone. *Computational Biology and Chemistry, 75,* 178–195.

[22] Harren, T., Gutermuth, T., Grebner, C., Hessler, G., & Rarey, M. (2024). Modern machine-learning for binding affinity estimation of protein–ligand complexes: Progress, opportunities, and challenges. *Wiley Interdisciplinary Reviews: Computational Molecular Science, 14*(3), e1716.

[23] Shen, C., Ding, J., Wang, Z., Cao, D., Ding, X., & Hou, T. (2020). From machine learning to deep learning: Advances in scoring functions for protein–ligand docking. *Wiley Interdisciplinary Reviews: Computational Molecular Science, 10*(1), e1429.

[24] Tapeh, A. T. G., & Naser, M. Z. (2023). Artificial intelligence, machine learning, and deep learning in structural engineering: a scientometrics review of trends and best practices. *Archives of Computational Methods in Engineering, 30*(1), 115–159.

[25] Yang, X., Wang, Y., Byrne, R., Schneider, G., & Yang, S. (2019). Concepts of artificial intelligence for computer-assisted drug discovery. *Chemical Reviews, 119*(18), 10520–10594.

[26] Bereau, T. (2021). Computational compound screening of biomolecules and soft materials by molecular simulations. *Modelling and Simulation in Materials Science and Engineering, 29*(2), 023001.

[27] Lu, W., Zhang, J., Huang, W., Zhang, Z., Jia, X., Wang, Z., ... & Zheng, S. (2024). DynamicBind: Predicting ligand-specific protein-ligand complex structure with a deep equivariant generative model. *Nature Communications, 15*(1), 1071.

[28] Zhang, Y., Luo, M., Wu, P., Wu, S., Lee, T. Y., & Bai, C. (2022). Application of computational biology and artificial intelligence in drug design. *International Journal of Molecular Sciences, 23*(21), 13568.

[29] *AI in drug discovery market size, share & trends [2028].* (2024). MarketsandMarkets. https://www.marketsandmarkets.com/Market-Reports/ai-in-drug-discovery-market-151193446.html

[30] Yang, J., Soltan, A. A., Eyre, D. W., Yang, Y., & Clifton, D. A. (2023). An adversarial training framework for mitigating algorithmic biases in clinical machine learning. *NPJ Digital Medicine, 6*(1), 55.

[31] Sehrawat, S. K. (2023). Transforming clinical trials: Harnessing the power of generative AI for innovation and efficiency. *Transactions on Recent Developments in Health Sectors, 6*(6), 1–20.

[32] Harrison, S. A., Allen, A. M., Dubourg, J., Noureddin, M., & Alkhouri, N. (2023). Challenges and opportunities in NASH drug development. *Nature Medicine, 29*(3), 562–573.

[33] Sefid Dashti, M. J., & Gamieldien, J. (2017). A practical guide to filtering and prioritizing genetic variants. *Biotechniques, 62*(1), 18–30.

[34] Pandey, M., Fernandez, M., Gentile, F., Isayev, O., Tropsha, A., Stern, A. C., & Cherkasov, A. (2022). The transformational role of GPU computing and deep learning in drug discovery. *Nature Machine Intelligence, 4*(3), 211–221.

Chapter 2

Techniques of AI/ML for Genomics Visualization in Plants

Amita Bisht, Diksha Dhiman and Abhilasha Chauhan

2.1 Introduction to Genomics Visualization

Genomics visualization plays a key role in interpreting biologically abundant data from genome sequencing and analysis. It includes methods and tools that transform complex genetic data into visual representations to help researchers understand the genomic structure, genetic interactions, and regulatory pathways. Tools that differ from nucleotide sequences to whole genomes allow the exploration of genomic data across scales and dimensions. This visual insight facilitates the identification of genetic variation, evolutionary relationships, and disease mechanisms and enables progress in fields such as biochemistry, agriculture, and environmental science.

2.1.1 Importance of Visualization in Plant Genomics

Visualization in plant genomics is the cornerstone of understanding the complexity of genetic information and translating this knowledge into practical applications. Genomic data, by its very nature, is extraordinarily complex and large, containing nucleotides, deep sequencing, multi-layered regulatory information, complex genes, proteins, and metabolic pathways. Effective visualization techniques are needed to make these complexities, including interactions, comprehensible enough to be easily analyzed and interpreted. Visual tools help visualize genomic sequences, compare genetic variation, and determine functional relationships of genomic elements. For

DOI: 10.1201/9781003617013-2

example, genome browsers allow researchers to traverse large genomic landscapes, visually identifying genes, regulatory regions, and structural changes with ease. These tools are essential to identify genes of interest that are responsible for specific traits, understand genetic diversity within and among plants, and explore their evolutionary relationships.

Furthermore, visualization facilitates the integration of disparate data sets, such as transcriptomics, proteomics, and metabolomics, which are essential for a comprehensive understanding of plant biology. Multi-omics data integration through visualization enables researchers to identify correlations and causal relationships at the molecular level. Important for identifying mechanisms of complex traits such as resistance or disease susceptibility For example, heat mapping plays a major role in determining gene expression profiles, allowing rapid identification of differentially expressed genes under different conditions. Our ability to visualize such datasets not only enhances our understanding of plant biology but also allows for the rapid breeding of new plant species with desirable traits and supports efforts for sustainable agriculture and food security.

Besides facilitating basic research, plant genetic engineering has important implications for applied science, especially in crop improvement and agricultural biotechnology. Assessment tools enable breeders and geneticists to make informed decisions in the selection of parent plants for breeding programs, increased yield, and nutrition for better crop growth with value and resilience to environmental stresses, for example. Tools that show quantitative trait loci (QTL) mapping results help identify genetic markers associated with beneficial traits, identify supported markers for selection, and accelerate breeding. In CRISPR and gene transfer, changes for other technologies and imaging tools help identify specific genomic targets for editing and facilitate plant creation.

Graphics also play an important role in communicating complex genomic data to multiple audiences, including policymakers, academics, and the public. Effective visual graphics can demystify the science of genomics, making it accessible to non-specialists, and it has been fascinating. This is especially important at a time when public understanding and acceptance of biotechnology can greatly influence policy decisions and funding allocations [1].

- ■ The Role of Visualization in Understanding Genomic Data
  Visualization plays an important role in understanding genomic data by transforming complex and high-resolution information into accessible objects, revealing patterns, relationships, insights, hidden sequences, analysis, and interpretation of genetic challenges. Genetic analysis techniques effectively enable researchers to decipher this complexity. Large genomic landscapes provide a graphical method of analysis, facilitating the identification of genes, regulatory regions, and structural variations in the genome. Heat maps serve to identify genes. Expressions at different levels under conditions revealing differential expression of genes reveal evolutionary relationships. Moreover,

interaction diagrams elucidate the interactions between genes and proteins, providing insight into the mechanisms underlying phenotypic traits.

By integrating and visualizing data from diverse sources such as transcriptomics, proteomics, and epigenomics, researchers can gain a mapping of a broader understanding of the genomic basis of complex traits and diseases that helps to generate and test hypotheses by highlighting anomalies and relationships that warrant further investigation. Furthermore, it enhances the communication of complex genomic findings to a wider audience, including scientists, policymakers, and the public, leading to greater understanding and contribution to genomic research. In summary, imaging is an indispensable tool in genomics, enabling usable knowledge translation in large and complex data sets. It facilitates progress in discovery and application [2].

■ Historical Perspectives on Genomics Visualization

Historical perspectives on genomics visualization emphasize the transformational journey from the basic level to sophisticated interactive tools necessary for modern genetic research. In the early days of genomics, data visualization consisted of charts and tables that only had a basic understanding of gene sequences and structures. The emergence of sequencing technologies during the decade, particularly the Sanger method of sequencing, expanded dramatically quantitative genetic data and required advanced methodological approaches to write things in order. These tools changed how scientists interpreted large genomic landscapes, including the identification of genes, regulatory elements, and structural changes if possible. In the 2000s, advances in sequencing method and high-level data further increased data complexity and volume, thus necessitating integrated dynamic imaging techniques. Today, genomic imaging tools are not only sophisticated but also accessible, AI. In addition to integrating machine learning (ML) to process big data to gain deeper insights into the genetic basis of disease, developmental biology, and functional genomics, imaging systems now support collaborative research, enabling scientists around the world to share and analyze genomic data in real time. The integration of multi-omics data visualization has further enhanced our understanding of complex biological systems. Looking ahead, the continued development of imaging tools promises to transform genomic research and personalized medicine. The diagram of the history of gene sequencing technology is shown in Figure 2.1.

2.2 Current Challenges in Genomics Visualization

Given the size and complexity of modern genomic data, genomic mapping faces several significant challenges. High-throughput sequencing generates large amounts of data that require advanced computational tools and processing power necessary for efficient imaging. Integrating diverse data types such as genomics,

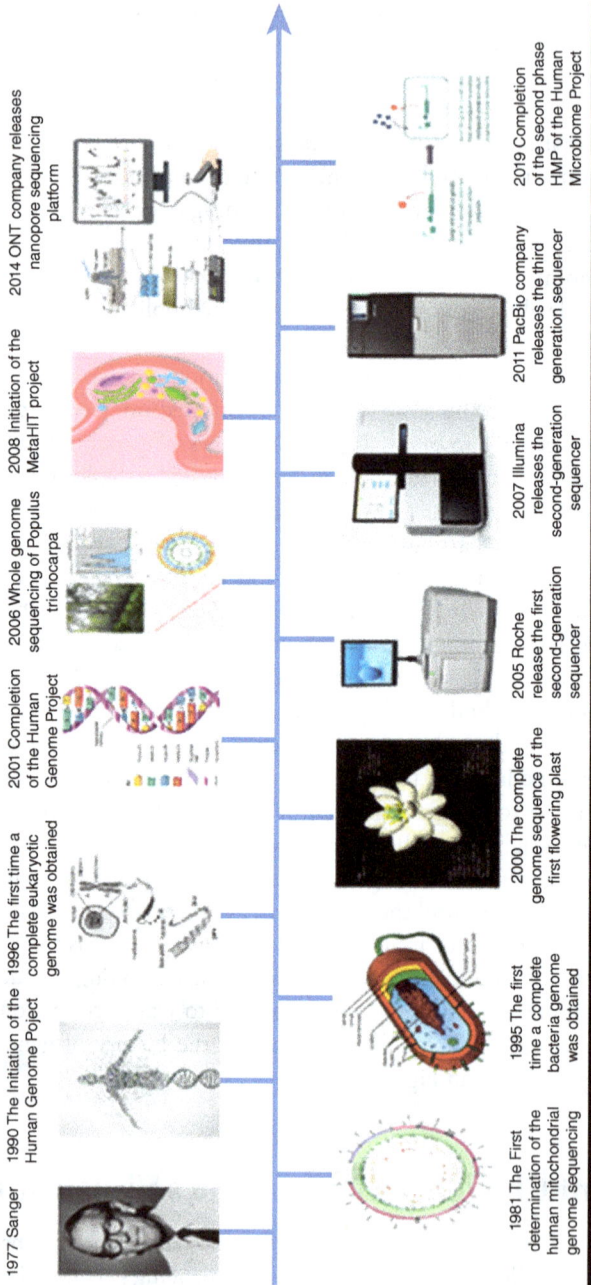

Figure 2.1   History of gene sequencing technology.

transcriptomics, and proteomics into visual system matching is difficult, often requiring sophisticated algorithms. Traditional linear representations struggle to capture complex genomic systems such as structural variants and gene fusions. There was a need for more advanced, often three-dimensional, visualization techniques and, because many tools are complex, and not user-friendly for non-specialists, there is a far more accessible interfaces. Data privacy and security concerns are becoming increasingly important, especially when genomics data are used in clinical settings. Finally, the rapidly evolving genomics technology requires frequent updating of imaging tools to remain relevant and effective. Addressing these challenges is essential to improving the understanding and use of genomic data [3, 4].

■ Complexity of Plant Genomes
Plant genomes exhibit incredible complexity due to their size, polyploidy (many chromosomes), and extensive sequence frequencies. Unlike simple organisms such as bacteria or yeast, plant genomes can consist of millions to millions of base pairs, in addition to many genes filled with non-coding regions. Plants frequently undergo genome duplication events throughout evolution, giving rise to genetic diversity and the possibility of internal modification in different environments. The presence of common elements presents challenges to genome assembly and annotation, making it difficult to identify functional elements and regulatory regions. Understanding the complexity of plant genomes is essential for crop improvement, biology conservation, and identifying the genetic basis of traits such as stress tolerance and disease resistance.

The volume and diversity of data pose significant challenges to genomics. The amount of data generated by modern sequencing technologies, typically terabytes per genome, requires complex computational infrastructure and efficient data management techniques on diverse features such as SNPs, CNVs, and the regulation of epigenetic modifications in populations and species. In addition to requiring advanced bioinformatics tools for integration with analysis, the integration of genomic data with other omics layers provides information. The difficulty is high, requiring careful integration and interpretation to yield meaningful insights. Control technologies require continuous innovation.

2.3 Impact of AI/ML on Genomics Visualization

AI/ML has revolutionized genomics visualization by enhancing data interpretation, enabling accurate analysis of complex genomic datasets, and facilitating the discovery of meaningful patterns and relationships. ML algorithms for data processing services are functional, such as feature extraction, pattern identification, and rapid genomic analysis. AI-powered tools such as deep learning models for genomic predictions are more accurate and enable advanced visualization techniques, such as 3D genome mapping and interactive data exploration. These innovations improve our understanding of genetics methods which is not only great but also identifies disease markers and optimizes treatment strategies. They also support personalized medicine and agricultural biotechnology through crop breeding programs by improving the quality.

- ■ Enhancements and Innovations
  Advances and innovations in genomics visualization are driven by technological advances, especially through the integration of AI/ML techniques. These innovations greatly improved the analysis and interpretation of complex genomic data. AI/ML algorithms enable efficient and accurate processing of large genomic datasets, automating tasks such as variant calling, genomic annotation, and pathway analysis. Deep learning models, such as convolutional neural networks (CNNs) and recurrent neural networks (RNNs), are complex models that remove correlation and transform the analysis of genomic data that are difficult to differentiate manually.

  Furthermore, AI-powered tools have facilitated the development of interactive and dynamic modeling techniques. These tools enable researchers to analyze genomic data in real time, visualize 3D genome structure, and explore spatial and temporal gene interactions. Such capabilities are essential for understanding the functional implications of genomic changes and regulatory elements.

  In addition, AI/ML has advanced predictive models in genomics, enabling the identification of genetic markers associated with complex diseases and traits. This predictive capability complements advances in precision medicine to develop therapeutic strategies based on the individual genomic profile for everyone.

  AI and ML have revolutionized genomics in many areas, showing impressive successes. AI algorithms in genomic variant calling have dramatically improved accuracy and performance in detecting genetic variants from sequencing data, critical to understanding disease pathways and underlying genetic diversity. ML models have predicted that drugs and target networks have accelerated the discovery of potential therapeutic agents and reduced development timelines [5].

2.4 Core AI/ML Techniques for Visualization

Major AI/ML techniques for visualization include deep learning, clustering, and dimension reduction, transforming any complex data sets into analytical eyes. CNNs and other deep learning models excel in image data manipulation and visualization, capture patterns and key reference group similar data points, and facilitate the identification of patterns and relationships across data sets. Dimensionality reduction techniques such as principal component analysis (PCA) and autoencoders simplify high-dimensional data, enabling clear visual representation and interpretation. All of these techniques combine to provide the ability to explore, analyze, and hear big data in science and utilities, which is huge.

2.5 Overview of AI/ML Concepts

The main AI/ML techniques for visualization in genomics include supervised and unsupervised learning methods. Supervised learning, such as decision trees and supporting interactive technologies, is used to perform classification tasks such as identifying disease markers from genomic data. Unsupervised learning, such as clustering algorithms, helps in identifying patterns in large datasets, and deep learning techniques, such as convolutional neural networks, help in gene expression analysis and genomic data exploration for image-based genomic visualization, so they do great, like 3D genome mapping. These techniques enable researchers to draw meaningful insights from complex genomic data, supporting advances in personalized medicine and agricultural and biological research.

AI: Artificial intelligence (AI) helps in data visualization and uses advanced algorithms to better identify interpretations of complex data sets. AI technology, etc., is powerful from the marks, which generate a scene of identical points upwards, neural networks of the high-dimensional data. Goridam uses this capability to enable AI to create interactive and insightful visualizations that aid in decision-making, data mining, and understanding of complex data structures. From trend recognition in economic data to biological interactions on the picture of difficulty.

ML: ML plays an important role in data visualization by stabilizing the interpretation and representation of complex datasets. ML algorithms facilitate the extraction of meaningful insights from data, enabling visualizations that reveal patterns, trends, and relationships. Devices such as clustering algorithms help to group similar data points, while PCA and t-distributed stochastic neighbor embedding (t-SNE). By automating data analysis and pattern recognition processes, ML enables the creation of interactive and dynamic models that support decision-making processes in a variety of industries, from business analytics to scientific research to healthcare services.

Types of Learning

■ **Supervised Learning**: Supervised learning is ML in which models are trained on labeled data. This means that each input in the training data set is associated with an output label, and the algorithm learns how to map the inputs to the correct output. The goal is to make this map general enough so that the model can make accurate predictions about new unobserved events. Typical applications include classification services, such as email spam detection, and regression services, such as predicting house prices. Supervised learning is increasingly used due to the simplicity of the procedure and the abundance of references in various fields.

■ **Unsupervised Learning**: Unsupervised learning involves training data structures without any label feedback. The algorithm attempts to find hidden patterns in the data. This indicator is particularly useful in operations in which the targets are compatible and for the purpose of eliminating the char numbers and simplifying the coal, as well as inspecting incompatible parts, or it is impossible.

■ **Reinforcement Learning**: Reinforcement learning is a form of ML in which an agent learns to make a decision by interacting with the environment. The agent receives feedback about rewards or punishments based on his actions and aims to maximize accumulated rewards over time. Unlike supervised learning, complete input–output pairs are not provided; instead, agents should analyze the consequences of their actions and learn from them. Reinforcement learning is widely used in applications that require sequential decision-making, such as sports games, robotics, and autonomous driving, where the goal is to develop strategies or systems that will produce better outcomes [6].

2.6 Machine Learning Algorithms for Visualization

ML algorithms greatly improve data visualization by enabling analysis and interpretation of complex data sets. Clustering algorithms, such as k-means and hierarchical clustering, insert similar data points to reveal patterns and relationships. Dimensionality reduction techniques, including PCA and t-distributed stochastic neighbor embedding (t-SNE), simplify high-dimensional data to lower dimensions, making it easier to check methods for detection anomalies, such as forest clearance, and are understood to reveal outlier contributions that may indicate significant deviations or errors. Furthermore, neural networks, especially CNNs, facilitate image development and analysis, resulting in detailed and insightful visual data. These systems collectively provide our visualization capabilities and improve our understanding of large, complex datasets.

2.7 Deep Learning Approaches

Deep learning techniques for visualization leverage the power of complex neural networks to extract and interpret complex patterns from data, increasing understanding and insight across tasks. CNNs are important for image-based visual processing, good for extraction, enabling applications like object detection and segmentation. RNNs excel in sequential data analysis, important for time series visualization and natural language processing applications, where time is very important for understanding dependencies. Transformers capture sequencing global dependencies in data and modify language structures and semantic functions, facilitating accurate and contextual representation of the data. These deep learning techniques provide extraction functions in which complex relationships are learned.

■ **Convolutional Neural Networks (CNNs)**: CNNs are vital in records visualization, especially in image and video processing. CNNs excel in getting to know scene functions sequentially from raw pixel statistics. Their framework includes convolutional layers that observe filters on the entered photo to stumble on features, which include edges, textures, and shapes, accompanied by means of pooling layers that reduce spatial dimensions at the same time as retaining crucial statistics. CNNs offer they're able to perform complicated and correct eye analysis and interpretation in fields that include laptop imaginative and prescient, medical imaging, and self-sustaining driving. The revolution did and caused the advent of equipment essential for complicated statistics visualization duties [7].

2.8 Visualization Techniques for Genomic Data

Techniques for genomic data include genome browsers for sequencing, heat maps for gene expression patterns, and grids for gene interactions. Tools such as the IGV and UCSC Genome Browser provide comprehensive genomic views, while Circos does the representation of genome variation in a circular array. These techniques transform complex genetic data into accessible data, helping to understand genetic structure, function, and relationships.

2.8.1 Sequence Data Visualization

Sequence data visualization techniques for genomic data include well-developed techniques for interpreting complex biological data. Genome browsers will continue to be foundational tools, providing interactive interfaces for genome sequencing, annotation, and advanced analysis. Heat mapping and cluster analysis elucidate biological processes and reveal gene expression in different conditions or tissues. Network visualization maps molecular interactions between genes, proteins, or regulatory elements and provides graphical insights into complex biological networks. Furthermore, 3D genome visualization techniques reveal the spatial structure and chromatin interactions necessary to understand gene regulation and genome architecture.

The systems integrated into the integrated model include several types of omics—genomics, transcriptomics, proteomics, and epigenomics. These techniques enable the efficient guidance of biological systems by incorporating molecular data into integrated visual images. Pathway discovery tools combine genomic data with metabolic pathways, revealing mechanistic relationships underlying diseases or traits. Interactive systems enhance analysis and interpretation, allowing users to visualize data, filter it, and easily integrate it with external data. These advanced techniques enable researchers to discover new biomarkers, elucidate biological pathways, and identify trends in advanced medicine, agriculture, and basic biological research.

■ Aligning and Visualizing DNA Sequences

The alignment and visualization of DNA sequences are vital for knowledge of genetic similarity, variation, and evolutionary relationships among organisms. Sequence alignment equipment, consisting of BLAST (Basic Local Alignment Search Tool), uses algorithms to evaluate nucleotide sequences, figuring out regions of homology or conservation. These styles seem, in a number of ways, along with pairs of matching sequences that highlight regions of concordance and dissimilarity between sequences. The tools extend this ability to compare more than two sequences simultaneously, revealing conserved patterns and evolutionary variation across species or across genomes. DNA sequence alignment mapping often affects nucleotide color coding for clarity, with distinctions indicating insertions or deletions in rows.

Advanced visualization tools combine assembly data with genomic annotations such as gene loci or regulatory elements to provide context for evolutionary studies or functional genomics research. Interactive visualization tools enable researchers to search for assemblies that it is dynamic, enlarging specific areas, and overlays with additional biological information for comprehensive analysis, facilitating research on pathogenic mutations and evolutionary history of organisms, from biomedical research to conservation biology, as needed for use in certain areas.

■ Visualization of Single Nucleotide Polymorphisms (SNPs)

The development of single nucleotide polymorphisms (SNPs) is important for understanding genetic variation and its impact in areas such as disease susceptibility, population genetics, and evolutionary biology. SNPs are the most common genetic variants that occur in individuals and are single nucleotide changes in the genome. The techniques used to generate SNPs help researchers identify, interpret, and analyze these changes in the genome.

Genome browsers such as the UCSC Genome Browser and Ensembl provide platforms for visualizing SNPs in their genomic context, allowing users to see their locations relative to SNP density plots of genes and other functional elements highlighting areas with high or low genetic variation, which can reveal the frequency and distribution of SNPs in different genomic regions. Heatmaps are another useful tool, enabling the visualization of SNP association data, such as linkage disequilibrium models, which predict non-random association of SNPs in populations.

Genome-wide association studies (GWAS) typically use Manhattan plots to visualize the significance of a genome-wide association. Each point on the plot represents an SNP, with its position on the x-axis so its genomic location and its y-axis kept consistent. In addition to the axis representation of the statistical significance of its association, tools such as the Integrative Genomics Viewer (IGV) offer great visualization capabilities, including zooming to specific SNPs. If you view sequences consistently and explore different explanations, it can link diversity to phenotypic traits and open insights into human health.

2.8.2 *Phylogenetic Analysis*

Phylogenetic analysis is an important tool in evolutionary biology that helps clarify evolutionary relationships between organisms or genes by comparing genetic, morphological, and biochemical data. The process begins with sequencing to identify conserved and variable regions in DNA, RNA, or protein sequences. The construction of these trees represents hypothesized evolutionary trajectories, with branch lengths indicating genetic distances and neurons identifying common ancestors. Visual tools such as MEGA and FigTree enhance the interpretation of these trees by detailed analysis of evolutionary relationships and annotations. This research is fundamental to studying species origins and diversity, understanding genetic diversity, and exploring the evolutionary history of life, providing important insights for fields ranging from genetics to conservation biology.

■ Constructing and Visualizing Phylogenetic Trees
Building and mapping phylogenetic trees are major trends in evolutionary biology, often providing insights into the evolutionary relationships between species or gene sequences. Phylogenetic trees begin with the alignment sequences and use DNA, RNA, or protein sequences to identify regions. These programs analyze sequence data to identify evolutionary pathways and create tree diagrams with branch lengths to identify genes of distances and branch points (nodes) representing common ancestors.

Mapping phylogenetic trees is important for the interpretation and determination of inferred evolutionary relationships. A variety of tools and software, such as MEGA, FigTree, and Dendroscope, provide a robust platform for visualizing these trees in a logical and understandable way, with root trees showing common ancestors or unrooted trees representing relationships that do not specify ancestral roots or patterns, or they can display interactive tree viewers for users to actively explore data, zoom in on specific branches, rotate the tree, and add additional information such as geographic classification or phenotypic traits together. These diagrams provide important insights into evolutionary processes, species, and biological genes.

◼ Integrating ML for Dynamic Tree Visualization 3.3 Heatmaps and Clustering
Integrating ML for dynamic tree modeling uses advanced methods to enhance
the analysis and correlation search of phylogenetic trees. ML methods can
analyze large datasets that tend to identify patterns and relationships that
mean building more accurate and informative trees. These dynamic visualizations allow users to interactively explore tree structure, modify findings, and
integrate additional data such as genetic and ecological data to gain deeper
insights into evolutionary relationships about how clustering algorithms can
group similar systems or species together to reveal evolutionary patterns and
differences. Heat maps can process information such as genetic variation or
expression levels, overlaying this information into a tree structure to provide a
comprehensive view of biological relationships and diversity. The combination
of dynamic ML and visualization tools empowers researchers to critically analyze and interpret complex family genetics. Integrating ML for dynamic tree
modeling uses advanced methods to enhance the analysis and correlation
search of phylogenetic trees. ML methods can analyze large datasets that tend
to identify patterns and relationships that mean building more accurate and
informative trees. These dynamic visualizations allow users to interactively
explore tree structure, modify findings, and integrate additional data such as
genetic and ecological data to gain deeper insights into evolutionary relationships about how clustering algorithms can group similar systems or species
together to reveal evolutionary patterns and differences. Heat maps can process information such as genetic variation or expression levels, overlaying this
information into a tree structure to provide a comprehensive view of biological relationships and diversity. The combination of dynamic ML and visualization tools empowers researchers to critically analyze and interpret complex
family genetics. Integrating ML for dynamic tree modeling uses advanced
methods to enhance the analysis and correlation search of phylogenetic trees.
ML methods can analyze large datasets that den to identify patterns and relationships that mean building more accurate and informative trees. This
dynamic visualization allows users to interactively explore tree structure,
exchange ideas, gain deeper insights into evolutionary relationships, and integrate new information such as genetic and ecological data so that clustering
algorithms can group similar systems or species together to reveal evolutionary
patterns and differences. Heat maps can process information such as genetic
variation or expression levels, overlaying this information on a tree structure
to provide a comprehensive view of biological relationships and diversity. The
combination of dynamic ML and visualization tools empowers researchers to
critically analyze and interpret complex family genetics.

◼ Creating Heatmaps for Gene Expression Data
Heat mapping for gene expression profiles is an important technique for visualizing relative levels of gene expression between samples or conditions. In this
way, the data are organized into graphs with rows representing genes and

columns representing samples. Each cell of the matrix is colored based on the expression of a gene in a particular sample, with horizontal colors indicating high, medium, and low expression levels, etc. Temperature images facilitate the identification of patterns and trends. Particularly valuable in large-scale studies, such as those involving microarray or RNA-seq data, where they help rapidly identify differentially expressed genes and evaluate the overall expression status by providing a simple and comprehensive visual summary; heat mapping enhances the ability to interpret complex gene expression and helps them advance research in areas such as genomics, oncology, and developmental biology.

■ Clustering Genomic Data with AI Techniques
Combining genomic data with AI techniques uses advanced algorithms to cluster similar genes or features, revealing biological structures and underlying structures. AI techniques such as k-means, hierarchical clustering, and more sophisticated deep learning techniques, which target genes with similar expression profiles, sequence homologies, or functional traits, or analyze large-scale genomic data sets to identify clusters of genomic regions These techniques can handle the complexity and high resolution of genomic data, effectively revealing meaningful patterns that may be overlooked by traditional methods of AI [8].

2.9 Advanced Visualization Techniques

Advanced visualization techniques in genomics include 3D genome mapping, which reveals the spatial arrangement of chromosomes; multi-omics integration, combining different types of data to identify complex biological relationships; and interactive dashboards that enable real-time analysis of genetic data.

2.9.1 3D Genomic Visualization

3-D genomic visualization is a powerful method that offers a three-dimensional example of genomic structures, permitting researchers to discover the spatial corporation and interactions within the genome. Unlike conventional linear visualizations, 3D fashions provide a more sensible perspective of the manner DNA is folded and packed in the nucleus, revealing the spatial proximity of far-off genomic areas and their regulatory interactions. This method is crucial for information on the complex architecture of chromatin, gene regulation, and the practical implications of genome enterprise. Techniques like Hi-C and different chromosome conformation seize techniques generate facts that may be visualized in 3D to map the interactions among first-rate additives of the genome. These visualizations assist in locating the structural foundation of gene regulation, becoming aware of chromosomal rearrangements related to illnesses, and offering insights into the dynamic nature of the genome in the cell context. By supplying a complete view of genomic structure, 3D visualization enhances our know-how of genetic law, genome features, and the underlying mechanisms of genetic issues.

■ Techniques for 3D Genome Mapping

3D genome mapping techniques include advanced techniques for capturing the spatial arrangement of the genome in the cell nucleus, providing a general view of how DNA regions interact in three dimensions. Key techniques include Hi-C, the use of proximity binding to measure the frequency of interactions between chromosome regions, thus creating a complete map of 3D genomic connectivity. Chromosome structure capture (3C) and its variables, for example, 4C and 5C, can also be used to identify linkages between specific genomic loci. These techniques yield reproducible 3D models of information and reveal how genes and regulators are placed relative to each other in atomic space. These 3D maps aid visualization basis of gene regulation, such as how distal enhancers affect gene expression and development. Three-dimensional genomes that provide insight into the spatial genomic organization underlying differentiation and disease will allow researchers to better understand the complex interplay between genomic structure and function.

■ Applications and Benefits in Plant Genomics

The use of 3D genome mapping in plant genomics is transforming our understanding of plant biology and reproduction. This approach allows researchers to examine the spatial structure of plant genes, providing insights into gene structure, chromatin structure, and interactions between genomic regions. 3D genome mapping helps identify regulatory factors and their target genes and elucidate the mechanisms of gene expression required for traits such as stress resistance, growth, and development. Understanding the 3D structure of the OM. In addition to genetic modifications and epigenetic modifications that contribute to the expression of desirable traits and improve resilient and high-yielding plant varieties, 3D genomic probes help to define complex genomes, and they provide a precise how-to genomics course. Overall, these applications are very useful in plant research by improving the understanding of genetic regulation, accelerating breeding programs, and contributing to sustainable agriculture and food security on the snow (Figure 2.2).

2.9.2 Network Visualization for Genomic Interactions

In network graphics for genomic networks, complex biological data are represented as networks, with nodes representing genomic elements such as genes or regulatory regions and edges indicating interconnections between them. It can add associations. Cytoscape and other network visualization tools allow researchers to create and visualize these networks, making it easier to identify regulatory genes, protein-protein interactions, and factors that change pathways. Researchers combine

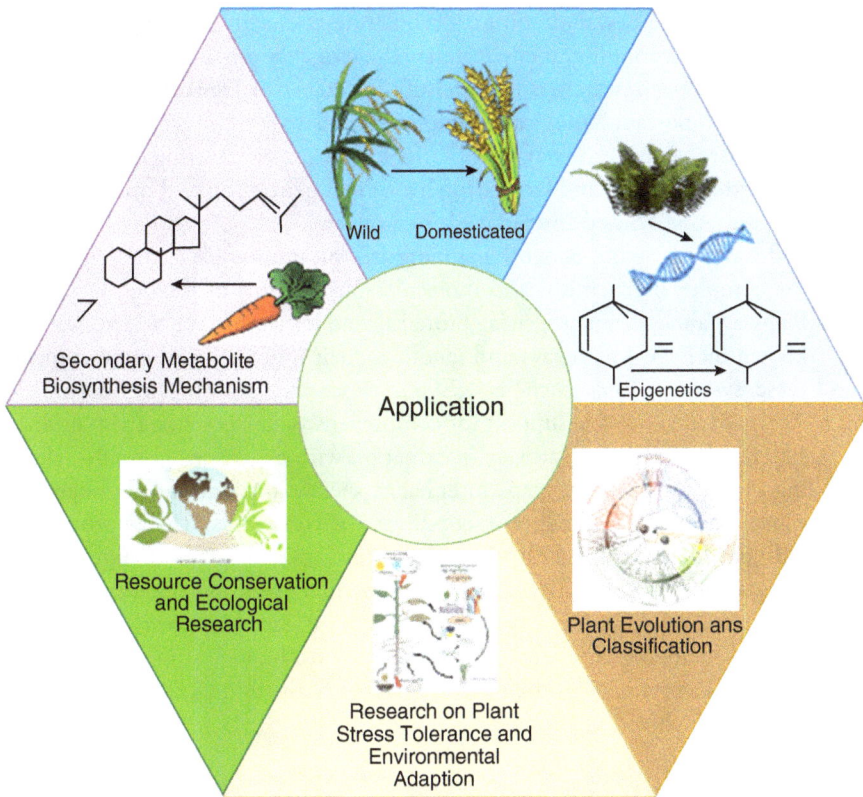

Figure 2.2 **Application of genetic sequencing technology.**

genomic data with network analysis key hubs (highly connected nodes that play important roles in biology) and identify modules (groups of tightly connected neurons). This approach helps to understand functional relationships between genomic elements, reveal regulatory mechanisms, and identify potential targets for medical applications or crop improvement in agriculture. Thus, network visualization gives us the ability to characterize genomic communications under more, advancing research in systems biology, biotechnology, and personalized medicine.

■ Visualizing Gene Networks
  Mapping gene interactions requires complex interactions and relationships between genes in biological systems. Gene networks are constructed based on experimental data such as gene expression, protein–protein interactions, and regulatory relationships. Visualization tools such as Cytoscape and Gephi enable researchers to visualize where nodes represent genes and edges show connections or relationships between them. These connections can reveal groups of genes or modules that work together in specific pathways or

biological processes, underpinning cellular functions, manifesting disease processes, and responding to environmental factors. By providing genetic insight into pathways, researchers can identify key genes or regulatory regions that regulate important biological functions, helping to identify biomarkers, therapeutic targets, and pathway possibilities for genetic engineering in biotechnology and agriculture and facilitating hypothesis generation and testing.

■ Pathway Analysis and Interactive Visualization

Pathway analysis and network mapping are important tools for understanding the complex biochemical and molecular mechanisms of biological systems. Pathway analysis maps genes, proteins, and other molecular entities into known biological pathways and identifies their functions and interactions in these systems. Tools such as KEGG, Reactome, and Ingenuity Pathway Analysis (IPA) provide support for comprehensive databases and visualization systems that integrate pathway information with experimental results, allowing the use of pathway maps to enhance specific interactions, highlight key veins, and visualize changes in conditions or treatments. This approach not only elucidates the functional relationships between different biomolecules but also helps to identify potential therapeutic targets and understand molecule mechanisms underlying diseases. By using flexible networks for search, network mapping facilitates deeper insights into biological mechanisms and identifies new targets for their involvement in health and biotechnology applications, which will accelerate.

2.9.3 *Temporal and Spatial Visualization*

Temporal and spatial analysis in biological research investigates how natural processes vary across time and space. Temporal analysis focuses on the dynamic nature of biological events, such as changes in gene expression during development, disease progression, or response to environmental factors, and reveals insights into the timing and sequence of molecular interactions. Techniques, along with pictures and spatial inscriptions, provide temporal and spatial elements, respectively. The integration of this research permits researchers to develop comprehensive models that capture the temporal evolution and spatial shape of biological structures, generating complex techniques such as tissue boom and cellular signaling pathways; its sickness approaches are profound.

■ Visualizing Temporal Changes in Gene Expression

Visualizing temporal changes in gene expression entails tracking and representing how gene activity varies over time under extraordinary conditions or developmental tiers. This process commonly employs time-series facts gathered through techniques like RNA sequencing or microarray analysis at a couple of time points. Visualization equipment inclusive of heatmaps, line graphs, and dynamic plots is used to demonstrate these adjustments, where every gene's expression degree is depicted throughout a temporal axis. For example, heatmaps can show fluctuations in expression by color-coding every gene's activity at different time durations, permitting patterns such as upregulation or downregulation to be easily determined. Line graphs or trend plots can, in addition, element the trajectories of precise genes through the years, highlighting responses to stimuli or development through organic cycles. Interactive visualization systems permit customers to explore those dynamic adjustments, offering insights into gene regulatory networks, identifying temporal biomarkers, providing information on the timing of gene expression occasions vital for procedures together with cellular differentiation, circadian rhythms, and disorder development. This complete visualization of temporal gene expression changes helps a deeper knowledge of the dynamic nature of genetic regulation and characteristics in numerous biological contexts.

■ Spatial Distribution and Mapping of Genomic Data
Spatial distribution and mapping of genomic information is the vicinity and interaction of genes with different genomic factors in bodily or cell surroundings. This technique affords insight into how gene expression and regulation range in specific tissues, organs, or cellular environments. Techniques together with spatial recording and in situ hybridization allow researchers to map gene interest immediately to tissue sections or mobile populations and monitor spatial patterns and gene expression dynamics. Advanced visualization tools and diagrams create special maps revealing the spatial relationships and incorporation of genomic information. Correlating genetic records with tissue improvement and organ features is important to information on complex biological procedures together with ailment pathology. If we take the spatial context of genomic statistics, it enables researchers to reveal the spatial dynamics of gene regulation, interaction, and useful heterogeneity in biological structures and offers deeper insights into the molecular foundation of health and ailment [8].

2.10 AI/ML Tools and Platforms for Visualization

AI and ML tools and visualization algorithms are empowering researchers to translate and analyze complex data into understandable visualizations. Tools like TensorFlow and PyTorch provide a robust framework for building deep learning models that can handle large amounts of data, enabling visualization and extraction of features necessary for visualization. Platforms like Tableau and D3.js for visualization advanced the ability to integrate with AI models to create dynamic and interactive graphics. Unique tools such as DeepLabCut provide identification and tracking of features in visual data, facilitating analysis of patterns and trends. These AI-enabled visualization technologies facilitate data mining large multidimensional systems and provide insights into data structures, relationships, and underlying patterns, where they are helping to visualize the complex relationships between genetic information and enable data-driven decision-making and innovation, in other areas such as finance, healthcare, and commerce.

2.10.1 Key Tools for Genomics Visualization

Specialized genomics visualization tools play an important role in the interpretation of complex genetic data by transforming it into accessible and informative visual methods. Tools such as the IGV and the UCSC Genome Browser provide access to analyze and visualize genomic data at specific genomic regions. Offering such features as zooming and integration of data types such as gene expression sequence variants, Cytoscape makes it easy to identify complex interactions and enables the identification of gene interactions and pathways. HiGlass is a key tool for high-resolution correlation matrix visualization of chromosome structure capture data, providing insight into the 3D structure of genomes. Furthermore, tools such as Circos provide the ability to spherically map a genome, images particularly useful for displaying genomic rearrangements and structural variations in genomics tools: Genomics is not necessary for research and allows scientists to efficiently analyze and interpret large genetic data, facilitating discovery in tasks such as functional genomics, developmental biology, and precision medicine.

- Overview of Popular Tools: TensorFlow, PyTorch, etc.
  TensorFlow and PyTorch are two of the most distinguished tools in the area of system studying and AI. TensorFlow, advanced with the aid of Google, is an open-source framework that excels in its flexibility and scalability, making it ideal for building and deploying deep getting-to-know models throughout a number of structures. It helps large operations on tensors and gives a complete surroundings, which includes TensorFlow Extended (TFX) for end-to-cease gadget mastering pipelines and TensorFlow Lite for deploying fashions on cellular and side devices. PyTorch, created by way of Facebook, is desired for its dynamic computation graph, which provides flexibility and simplicity of use, particularly in study settings. Its intuitive interface and robust network assist make it a popular choice for fast prototyping and experimentation. PyTorch is fantastically valued for responsibilities that require frequent changes to the community architecture during development. Both frameworks guide an extensive variety of applications, from pc imaginative and prescient to herbal language processing, and combine well with other tools and libraries, using improvements in AI and deep learning.
- Features and Capabilities
  The features and capabilities of TensorFlow and PyTorch make them powerful tools for ML and deep learning. TensorFlow provides a flexible and scalable framework that supports a wide range of applications on multi-dimensional arrays (tensors) and is comprehensive with TensorFlow Extended (TFX) for complete ML pipeline management, TensorFlow Lite for mobile embedded

devices. Deployed ecosystem implementation, and TensorFlow.js for browser-based ML. It also provides strong support for high-level APIs like Keras, which makes architecture sampling easier, and also provides strong support for low-level APIs for more granular control. PyTorch, on the other hand, is known for its dynamic computer graph, which allows for real-time network analysis, making it particularly suitable for analysis and prototyping. PyTorch's easy-to-understand syntax and strong support for fast GPU delivery facilitate the complex development of neural networks. Both frameworks facilitate seamless integration with other libraries and tools such as NumPy and SciPy and support advanced ML tasks such as natural language processing, image and video recognition, and wearable learning intensify and raise the importance of academic and industrial AI applications [9]

2.10.2 Integration with Genomic Databases

The integration of TensorFlow and PyTorch into genomic databases enhances their usefulness in bioinformatics and genomics research. This framework provides strong support for processing large genomic data through seamless integration with popular genomic databases such as NCBI GenBank and NSEMBL and the flexibility of the UCSC Genome Browser TensorFlow to enable researchers to take the lead efficiently process, analyze, and access genomic data using its extensive computing capabilities and distributed resources. Visualization can also us PyTorch. Its dynamic computing graph and GPU acceleration accelerate data processing and modeling performance, making it ideally suited for complex genomic analyzes and deep learning applications. The use of these systems enables researchers to explore biological datasets intensively, open insights into genetic variation, regulatory mechanisms, and disease pathways in genomics, provide the ability to address important challenges, such as species discovery, gene expression analysis, and personalized medicine, leading to advances in understanding and treatment of genetic disorders and diseases.

■ Combining AI/ML Tools with Genomic Data Repositories
  Combining AI/ML tools with genomic data repositories transforms bioinformatics by using advanced algorithms to extract meaningful insights from large sets of genomic data. Tools like TensorFlow and PyTorch and repositories like NCBI GenBank and ENSEMBL integrate to provide efficient data preprocessing and feature extraction, and enable predictive modeling. This framework enables researchers to tackle complex challenges such as variant calling, gene expression profiling, genotype-phenotype correlations, and more; handle new AI/ML tools by automating data interpretation and increasing computational efficiency in genetics and personalized medicine of the Yomarker; facilitate the discovery of therapeutic targets and genomic signatures; and pave the way for more accurate diagnosis and customized treatment in health and biotechnology.

■ Practical Integration Examples
Practical examples of AI/ML tools and genomic data storage include applications in genomic bioinformatics; for example, researchers can use TensorFlow
or PyTorch to model deep learning of gene function based on sequence data
from repositories such as ENSEMBL or GenBank. These models can classify
gene mutations, identify disease-associated mutations, or predict protein
structure and function to aid in drug discovery and personalized medicine.
Furthermore, AI-powered tools can enable the automated analysis of large sets
of genomic data for regulatory elements, gene interactions, and developmental patterns if identification is enabled. Such integration simplifies data interpretation processes, accelerates analysis, and enhances our understanding of
complex biological systems, ultimately contributing to advances in genomic
medicine and agriculture.

2.10.3 Custom Visualization Solutions

Information visualization solutions in genomics use customized techniques to efficiently display and interpret complex biological data. These solutions often require
specialized software development or modification of existing tools to meet specific
research needs. For example, custom scripts or applications can integrate with
genomic databases to map individual genomic profiles, gene expression patterns, or
chromosome interactions. Interactive interfaces enable researchers to dynamically
explore data and modify parameters and visual representations to reveal patterns or
reveal hidden relationships. Such solutions also enable the integration of diverse data
types such as genomic sequences, epigenetic markers, and clinical metadata to facilitate comprehensive analysis and hypothesis generation. Optimizing visualization
tools enables researchers to address genomics' unique challenges.

■ Developing Tailored Visualization Tools
Visual tools designed for genomics involve building customized software solutions to address specific research goals and complex data in biology. These
tools are designed to visualize genomic data and have been interpreted in ways
that are not supported by available standard software. These development processes typically start with specific requirements for genealogical data, such as
complex genetics and local geographic connections, and then researchers and
developers work together. Where the skeleton is for the cry, Jum- Add interactive elements for making and comparative analysis These tools can integrate
with genomic databases and use advanced visualization techniques, such as
3D rendering for spatial genomics or grid graphs enable gene regulatory networks to enhance understanding of data, accelerate discovery, and introduce
scientists' visualization tools. Introduce biological mechanisms that drive linear mutations, disease mechanisms, and evolutionary relationships under the
Deeper You can gain insight [10].

2.11 AI/ML-Enhanced Visualization Workflows

AI/ML-enhanced visualization workflow refers to the integration of AI and ML techniques in the visualization process of complex data, especially in genomics, healthcare, finance, and other areas. So that researchers can gain meaningful insights and make data-driven decisions.

2.11.1 Data Pre-processing and Transformation

Effective visualization in genomic data analysis relies on careful data pre-processing and transformation procedures. This section explores the foundational steps needed to prepare data for analytical visualization.

- Data Cleaning and Normalization
  Genomic datasets frequently comprise noise and inconsistencies, which can obscure meaningful patterns. AI and device mastering algorithms play a pivotal function in automating statistics cleansing methods, identifying outliers, and ensuring record integrity. Through superior statistical strategies and sample popularity, these algorithms streamline the coaching phase, improving the satisfaction and reliability of subsequent visualizations.
- Feature Extraction and Selection
  Once facts are cleaned and normalized, the venture shifts to extracting relevant functions and deciding on those which can be maximum informative for visualization. Machine getting-to-know techniques, which include dimensionality discount, clustering, and feature importance analysis, help in identifying key genomic attributes. These extracted capabilities serve as the constructing blocks for growing insightful, visible representations that facilitate deeper insights into genetic information.

2.11.2 Visualization Pipeline Design

Visualization pipeline layout refers to the method of making and enforcing a chain of steps that remodels raw information into meaningful visible representations. In the context of AI/ML, more advantageous visualization workflows and visualization pipeline design include integrating system mastering algorithms and advanced visualization strategies to optimize how facts are processed and offered visually.

- Designing AI-Driven Visualization Pipelines
  AI-pushed visualization pipelines combine gadget-studying models with interactive visualization gear to give genomic information in an understandable format. These pipelines leverage strategies, which include neural networks for sample recognition, selection trees for type, and deep-gaining knowledge

for photo analysis. By combining those technologies, researchers can find hidden patterns and correlations within big genomic datasets [11].

■ Tools and Techniques for Pipeline Implementation
A variety of different tools and techniques support AI-powered visualization pipelines. From specialized software platforms to customized algorithms, these features empower researchers to create custom solutions that meet the unique challenges of genomic data visualization. Visualization libraries such as D3.js and Plotly complement interactive visualization frameworks such as TensorFlow and PyTorch and the boards enable seamless integration of models for prediction.

2.11.3 Automation of Visualization Tasks

Automation represents a transformative frontier in genomic data visualization, reducing human intervention and increasing productivity and scalability. This section explores the application and implications of automating visualization tasks.

■ Automating Genomic Data Visualization with AI
Automation of genomic data visualization uses AI and ML algorithms to rapidly analyze and interpret complex biological data. By focusing more on common tasks such as data parsing, feature extraction, and visual generation, researchers can focus more on hypothesis generation and scientific discovery. Moreover, AI-powered algorithms change over time, making visual representations based on changing data sets more accurate and relevant [12].

■ Benefits and Challenges
While automation brings significant benefits, including faster analysis and repeatability, it also comes with challenges. These include algorithmic bias, the ability to automate the interpretation of results, and the need for a robust validation framework. Addressing these challenges is essential to realizing the full potential of genomic data automation in research and clinical applications.

2.12 Case Studies and Real-World Applications

2.12.1 Functional Genomics and Gene Prediction

Functional genomics investigates the role of genes in biology, while genomic prediction identifies gene locations and functions in the genome. This section explores how AI and ML are revolutionizing the mapping of gene function and interaction networks [13].

■ AI/ML in Gene Function Analysis
Advances in AI enable comprehensive analysis of gene function by combining multi-omic data with the prediction of gene interactions. Visualizing these

interactions through interactive diagrams and interaction diagrams elucidates complex biological mechanisms, providing insights into disease mechanisms and therapeutic targets [14].

■ Visualization of Gene Networks and Interactions
   Graph-based tools such as Cytoscape and Gephi visualize gene interactions, focusing on regulatory interactions and pathway interactions. ML algorithms streamline network calculations, allowing researchers to identify new gene associations and biomarkers important for precision medicine [15].

2.12.2 Crop Improvement and Genomic Selection

In agricultural genomics, AI-driven visualization tools facilitate the breeding of resilient plants through facts-pushed decision-making and precision agriculture techniques [15].

Table 2.1   Comparison Table: Visualization Tools in Functional Genomics

Visualization Tool	Features	Applications	Benefits
Cytoscape	Network visualization, pathway analysis	Gene function analysis, regulatory network exploration	Detailed visualization of gene interactions and pathways. Allows for customization with plugins for particular analyses inclusive of protein–protein interplay networks (PPIs).
Gephi	Graph visualization, community detection	Network analysis, protein–protein interaction networks	Support large graph images, local detection, and planning algorithms for robust network analysis. It enables the interactive analysis of gene interactions and community structures [14].

Table 2.2 Comparison Table: AI Techniques in Crop Genomics

AI Technique	Applications	Benefits	Challenges
Machine Learning	Genomic selection, phenotype prediction	Improved breeding efficiency, trait optimization	Data quality, model interpretability
Deep Learning [15]	Image analysis, genotype–phenotype mapping	Automated feature extraction, accuracy in complex data	Computational resources, training time

- Visual Tools for Plant Breeding
  AI-enhanced visualization tools support phenotype analysis, genotype–phenotype mapping, and marker-assisted selection. By integrating genomic data with the environment, researchers are improving crop yields, disease resistance, and nutrient value through targeted breeding programs.
- Applications in Crop Genomics
  The case studies illustrate the application of AI in crop genomics from GWAS to genomic selection. Visualizing genomic landscapes allows breeders to identify beneficial alleles and accelerates the development of climate-tolerant crop varieties [16].

2.12.3 Comparative Genomics and Evolutionary Studies

Comparative genomics examines genetic similarities and differences between species, providing insights into evolutionary processes and species diversity.

- Visualizing Genomic Similarities and Differences
  AI-powered comparative genomics tools compare genomes at scale, revealing evolutionary relationships and adaptive traits. Visualization techniques such as genome alignment and phylogenetic trees reveal genomic synthesis and structural changes important for evolutionary analysis [17].
- Case Studies on Evolutionary Analysis
  From ancient DNA reconstruction to population genomics, AI-enabled imaging transforms complex genomic data into evolutionary data. The case studies highlight success in understanding species events, migration patterns, and adaptive evolution across classes.

2.13 Future Trends and Challenges in AI/ML Visualization

2.13.1 Emerging Trends in AI/ML for Genomics

The future of AI/ML in genomics visualization is shaped by ongoing innovation and interdisciplinary collaboration.

■ Latest Innovations and Research Directions
  Advances in translational AI, integrated learning, and single-cell genomics are redefining how researchers analyze and visualize complex biological data. The combination of AI with quantum computing promises unprecedented computational power for genomic simulation and personalized medicine.
■ Predictive Models and Visualization Techniques
  Next-generation sequencing and spatial registration technologies are driving demand for predictive models and visualization techniques that can handle multiple datasets. AI interprets large genomic data and predicts disease risk and treatment outcomes with high accuracy. There is nothing.

2.13.2 Challenges and Considerations

Despite its transformative potential, AI/ML-driven genomic visualization faces inherent challenges that require careful consideration and ethical scrutiny.

■ Technical Challenges: Data Volume, Algorithm Complexity
  Managing big-scale genomic datasets necessitates scalable AI architectures and statistics storage solutions. Addressing algorithmic complexity and computational performance ensures well-timed record evaluation and actual-time choice-making in medical settings.
■ Ethical and Privacy Issues in Genomic Data Visualization
  Protecting genomic privacy and reducing biases in AI algorithms are paramount. Ethics protocols promote transparency and patient consent in genomic research and health care and guide responsible data use.

2.13.3 Future Directions

2.13.3.1 Future Directions: Potential Developments and Innovations

AI/ML advances in genomics visualization promise transformative developments that will reshape scientific research and agricultural practices in the coming years:

■ Potential Developments and Innovations

1. **Integration of Quantum Computing**: Quantum computing has the potential to revolutionize genomic data analysis by dramatically accelerating complex computations. By harnessing the principles of quantum computing, algorithms can increase the accuracy and scalability of genomic analysis, allowing researchers to overcome previously insurmountable challenges in data handling and processing in the picture.

2. **Personalized Genomics and Healthcare**: AI-driven genomic visualization will enable personalized medicine strategies based on individual genetic profiles. The integration of genomic data with clinical outcomes and environmental factors will facilitate accurate diagnosis, treatment selection, and prevention strategies tailored to each patient's unique genetic profile.

3. **Real-time Data Analysis**: Advances in AI algorithms and cloud computing infrastructure will enable real-time analysis of streams of genomic data. This capability is particularly important in areas such as communicable disease surveillance and outbreak prediction, where timely genomic insights can inform public health interventions and strategies to prevent the sighting.

4. **Ethical and Regulatory Frameworks**: As the application of AI/ML in genomics expands, stronger ethical guidelines and regulatory frameworks will be needed to ensure responsible data use, privacy protection, and access to genomic technologies exactly.

■ Impact on Plant Science and Agricultural Research

The integration of AI/ML into plant genomics visualization is set to transform several fundamental aspects of agricultural practices and scientific research:

Table 2.3   Potential Applications of Quantum Computing in Genomics

Application	Description
Genome Assembly and Simulation	Quantum algorithms can boost the assembly of complicated genomes and simulate molecular interactions with extraordinary velocity.
Drug Discovery and Personalized Medicine	Quantum computing enables specific modeling of molecular interactions, facilitating drug discovery and customized remedy techniques.
Genomic Data Encryption	Quantum encryption strategies beautify genomic facts security and privacy, protecting touchy statistics from unauthorized get entry.

Table 2.4 Impact of AI/ML on Precision Agriculture

Impact Area	Description
Genomic Selection	AI-pushed genomic choice enhances breeding performance with the aid of predicting tendencies from genomic data.
Disease Management	Predictive models help in the early detection and control of crop diseases, optimizing yield.
Environmental Sustainability	Precision agriculture minimizes aid use and reduces environmental impact through records-pushed practices.
Crop Resilience to Climate Change	AI identifies genetic tendencies for climate resilience, developing plants suitable to changing environmental conditions.

■ Impact Areas
  - **Precision Agriculture**: AI-driven genomic tools will optimize crop breeding programs by linking genetic markers to desirable traits such as yield potential, disease resistance, and nutrition. Precision agricultural techniques will enable farmers to make data-driven decisions to reduce environmental impact and increase productivity.
  - **Climate Resilience**: Predictive models and genomic insights play an important role in developing climate-resistant crop varieties that can thrive in changing environments. AI algorithms will help identify genetic variation and modify agricultural practices accordingly to control them and predict and mitigate climate change impacts on agriculture.
  - **Global Food Security**: By improving crop yields, resilience, and nutritional value, AI-powered genomics will help advance global food security. Innovative approaches to animal husbandry and sustainable agriculture supported by AI technology will enable farmers to meet the growing demand for nutritious food in a world of limited resources.

2.14 Summary and Conclusions

2.14.1 Key Takeaways

Recap of AI/ML Techniques for Genomics Visualization: This chapter examined the transformative impact of AI and ML techniques on visualization of genomic data. From pre-processing to modeling to visualization tools and predictive analytics, AI is increasing the ability of researchers to derive mean-ingful insights from complex biological data.

Summary of Case Studies and Applications: Developments in functional genomics, crop breeding, and comparative genomics demonstrate the versatil-ity and applicability of AI/ML in biological research. Tools such as Cytoscape and Gephi enable the visualization of genetic networks, while deep learning models advance genotype–phenotype mapping and disease prediction.

2.14.2 Final Thoughts: The Future of AI/ML in Plant Genomics Visualization

Looking ahead, the convergence of AI/ML and plant genomics visualization holds profound implications for agricultural innovation, sustainable development, and global food security. As this technology evolves, it promises to pave the way for unprecedented advances in how we understand, analyze, and manipulate genetic information in plants, in agricultural practices, and beyond.

Advancements in Agricultural Productivity and Sustainability

AI/ML-powered genomics visualization is poised to increase agricultural productiv-ity by enabling more accurate and efficient crop breeding strategies. Researchers, nutritional indicators, etc., are able to identify genealogical characters with desired traits such as generation, increase disease resistance of new crops, and enhance resis-tance. It also reduces its dependence on the shell.

In addition, the AI/ML framework facilitates the prediction of plant responses to environmental factors, enabling the development of priority measures to reduce crop losses and maximize resource utilization as well. Precision agricultural practices informed by real-time genomic insights reduce water use, fertilizer use, and green-house gas emissions and promote agricultural practices.

Unlocking New Discoveries and Addressing Global Challenges

The integration of AI/ML into plant genomics visualization holds the promise of unlocking new biological approaches and accelerating scientific discovery. By deciphering complex genetic networks and regulatory interactions, researchers can uncover the molecular mechanisms underlying plant growth, disease resis-tance, and stress tolerance. This insight does not provide the basic understanding we have of plant biology but is not only profound but also informs the develop-ment of new biotechnological solutions to improve crop traits and agricultural outcomes.

Ethical and Regulatory Considerations

As AI/ML technologies transform plant genomics research, issues such as data privacy, consent, and intellectual property rights related to genomic data ownership need to be carefully considered and controlled to create an ethical and legal framework for it. These developments have been ensured to be implemented responsibly and with precision. To overcome these ethical challenges and maintain public confidence in genomic research and its applications, transparent communication and cooperation between researchers, policymakers, and stakeholders are essential.

Conclusion: A Transformative Frontier in Scientific Research

In conclusion, AI/ML-pushed genomics visualization represents a transformative frontier of medical research and gives exceptional opportunities to improve our knowledge of genetics and for agricultural practices to take off, enhance, and beautify global meal security. Using the intersection of AI/ML algorithms, quantum computing, non-public genomics, and ethical concerns, researchers can deal with the complicated challenges dealing with agriculture and society. This combination guarantees no longer alternating crop production and consumption but additionally makes contributions to sustainable improvement dreams and improves human fitness and well-being globally. Even the electricity gradually down takes place. As we embody this technology, there is first-rate capability for innovation, collaboration, and high-quality impact inside the field of destiny plant genomics and beyond.

References

[1] Sofi, Parvaze A., et al. (2024). Decoding life: Genetics, bioinformatics, and artificial intelligence. In *A Biologist s Guide to Artificial Intelligence*. Academic Press, 47–66.
[2] Walsh, Jason John, Mangina, Eleni, & Negrão, Sonia. (2024). Advancements in imaging sensors and AI for plant stress detection: A systematic literature review. *Plant Phenomics*, 6, 0153.
[3] Alam, Shabroz, Israr, Juveriya, & Kumar, Ajay. (2024). Artificial intelligence and machine learning in bioinformatics. In *Advances in Bioinformatics*. Singapore: Springer Nature Singapore, 321–345.
[4] Islam, Sumaiya, et al. (2024). Machine vision and artificial intelligence for plant growth stress detection and monitoring: A review. *Precision Agriculture*, 6(1), 34.
[5] Naik, Yogesh Dashrath, et al. (2024). Bioinformatics for plant genetics and breeding research. In *Frontier Technologies for Crop Improvement*. Singapore: Springer Nature Singapore, 35–64.
[6] Dhakshayani, J., Surendiran, B., & Jyothsna, J. (2024). Artificial intelligence in precision agriculture: A systematic review on tools, techniques, and applications. *Predictive Analytics in Smart Agriculture*, 37–57.

[7] Hu, Haifei, et al. (2024). Plant pangenomics, current practice and future direction. *Agriculture Communications*, 100039.

[8] Sudarsanan, Valsala, Kumar, Suvanish, & Sreekumar, Nidhin. (2024). Bioinformatic resources for plant genomic research. *Current Bioinformatics* 19(6), 513–529.

[9] Guenzi-Tiberi, Pierre, et al. (2024). LocoGSE, a sequence-based genome size estimator for plants. *Frontiers in Plant Science*, 15, 1328966.

[10] Kuan Ho, Wai, et al. (2024). A genomic toolkit for winged bean Psophocarpus tetragonolobus. *Nature Communications*, 15, 1901.

[11] Sboner, A., Mu, X. J., Greenbaum, D., & Gerstein, M. (2011). The real cost of sequencing: Higher than you think!. *Genome Biology*, 12(8), 125. doi: 10.1186/gb-2011-12-8-125

[12] Gehlenborg, N., O'Donoghue, S. I., Baliga, N. S., Goesmann, A., Hibbs, M. A., Kitano, H., … & Sansone, S. A. (2010). Visualization of omics data for systems biology. *Nature Methods*, 7(3 Suppl), S56–S68. doi:10.1038/nmeth.1436

[13] Shannon, P., Markiel, A., Ozier, O., Baliga, N. S., Wang, J. T., Ramage, D., … & Ideker, T. (2003). Cytoscape: A software environment for integrated models of biomolecular interaction networks. *Genome Research*, 13(11), 2498–2504. doi: 10.1101/gr.1239303

[14] Bastian, M., Heymann, S., & Jacomy, M. (2009). Gephi: An open source software for exploring and manipulating networks. *International AAAI Conference on Weblogs and Social Media*. Retrieved from: https://gephi.org/publications/gephi-bastian-feb09.pdf

[15] LeCun, Y., Bengio, Y., & Hinton, G. (2015). Deep learning. *Nature*, 521(7553), 436–444. doi: 10.1038/nature14539

[16] Krzywinski, M., Schein, J., Birol, I., Connors, J., Gascoyne, R., Horsman, D., … & Marra, M. A. (2009). Circos: An information aesthetic for comparative genomics. Genome research, 19(9), 1639–1645. doi:10.1101/gr.092759.109

[17] Park, Y., & Yun, J. Y. (2021). A design case study of artificial intelligence pipeline visualization. *Archives of Design Research*, 34(1), 133–155.

Chapter 3

Computing Architectures on the Cloud to Address Current Problems in Structural Bioinformatics

Diksha Dhiman and Amita Bisht

3.1 Introduction to Structural Bioinformatics

3.1.1 Overview of Structural Bioinformatics

Specialized in bioinformatics, structural bioinformatics studies and forecasts huge three-dimensional biological structures, including complexes, proteins, and nucleic acids. The field uses computational tools and techniques to understand the spatial arrangement and interactions of the atoms in these macromolecules [1]. The primary objectives of structural bioinformatics include:

- **Structure Prediction**: Prediction of 3D structures of macromolecules from their amino acid or nucleotide sequences.
- **Molecular Dynamics (MD)**: The physical motions of atoms and molecules can be simulated over time to understand their stability and interaction.
- **Function Annotation**: Measurement of the biological activity of macromolecules based on their structure.
- **Drug Design**: Identification of potential drug targets based on interactions with biological macromolecules and optimization of drug molecules.

DOI: 10.1201/9781003617013-3

3.1.2 Importance in Modern Biology and Medicine

Structural bioinformatics is pivotal in modern biology and medicine for several reasons:

- **Drug Discovery and Development**: By understanding the 3D structure of proteins and other macromolecules, researchers can develop more effective and specific drugs, reducing the time and costs associated with drug development.
- **Understanding Disease Mechanisms**: Systematic insights into how mutations affect protein function can elucidate the molecular basis of diseases, helping to develop targeted therapies.
- **Biotechnology and Synthetic Biology**: Knowledge of macromolecular structures enables the design of proteins and nucleic acids with desired properties for industrial biomedical applications.
- **Personalized Medicine**: Structural bioinformatics can contribute to personalized medicine by showing how individual genetic variations affect protein structure and function, resulting in personalized medicine.

3.1.3 Challenges in Structural Bioinformatics

Despite its significant contributions, structural bioinformatics faces several challenges:

- **Computational Complexity**: Predicting and modeling the structure of large macromolecules requires extensive computational resources.
- **Data Integration**: Combining structural information with other biological information, such as genomic and proteomic data, is challenging but necessary for comprehensive analysis.
- **Accuracy and Reliability**: Verifying the accuracy of computer predictions and assumptions is critical, as mistakes can lead to incorrect conclusions.
- **Scalability**: Structural bioinformatics studies require scalable and efficient computer systems to handle the volume of data generated.

3.1.4 The Role of Computing Architectures

Computer systems play an important role in solving the challenges of structural bioinformatics. They provide the computing power, storage, and tools needed for complex research and large-scale design. Traditional computing infrastructure, such as on-premises servers and high-performance computing (HPC) clusters, has been essential to the industry's growth, but the advent of cloud computing offers new opportunities for scalability, cost efficiencies, and access to the means of obtaining [2].

3.2 Fundamentals of Cloud Computing

3.2.1 What Is Cloud Computing?

The delivery of computer services via the Internet (the "cloud"), including servers, storage, databases, networking, software, and analytics, is known as cloud computing. These services let customers pay only for consumables and offer flexibility, quick innovation, and affordability [3] (Figure 3.1).

Key Characteristics of Cloud Computing

- **On-Demand Self-Service**: Without assistance from the service provider, users are able to allocate processing power automatically as needed.
- **Widespread Network Access**: Since cloud services are web-based and can be accessed via a standard method, using them across devices is encouraged.
- **Resource pooling**: On demand, cloud providers can dynamically assign and re-provision resources by pooling their computer resources to service many consumers.
- **Rapid Elasticity**: In response to consumer needs, products can be released at scale and supplied with ease and speed.
- **Measured Service**: By using metering capabilities, cloud systems automatically regulate and optimize resource utilization, fostering transparency between the supplier and the customer.

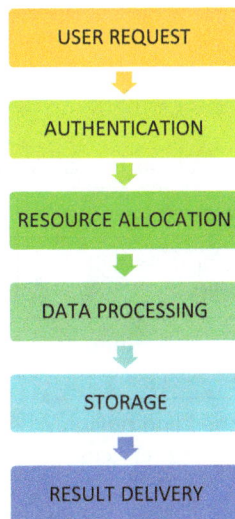

```
┌─────────────────────┐
│    USER REQUEST     │
└─────────────────────┘
          ⬇
┌─────────────────────┐
│   AUTHENTICATION    │
└─────────────────────┘
          ⬇
┌─────────────────────┐
│ RESOURCE ALLOCATION │
└─────────────────────┘
          ⬇
┌─────────────────────┐
│   DATA PROCESSING   │
└─────────────────────┘
          ⬇
┌─────────────────────┐
│       STORAGE       │
└─────────────────────┘
          ⬇
┌─────────────────────┐
│   RESULT DELIVERY   │
└─────────────────────┘
```

Figure 3.1   Cloud Computing Process.

3.2.2 Key Components of Cloud Infrastructure

The essential elements of cloud infrastructure consist of [4]:

- **Compute Power**: Virtual machines (VMs), containers, and serverless computing applications that enable scalable processing.
- **Storage**: Scalable and flexible storage solutions for managing large amounts of data, such as object storage, file storage, and block storage.
- **Networking**: A fast and reliable network service that allows data to be transferred in and between clouds.
- **Services and APIs**: Application programming interfaces (APIs) that provide core functionality, such as machine learning (ML), data analysis, and security.

3.2.3 Cloud Service Models (IaaS, PaaS, and SaaS)

Cloud services are categorized into three primary models:

- **Infrastructure as a Service (IaaS)**: It offers networking, storage, and virtualized hardware resources like VMs. Users are not accountable for maintaining the underlying infrastructure; they only have authority over operating systems and apps. Azure VMs and AWS EC2 are two examples [5].
- **Platform as a Service (PaaS)**: With the help of its middleware and development mechanisms, developers can build and run apps without worrying about maintaining the supporting infrastructure. AWS Elastic Beanstalk and Google App Engine are two examples [6].
- **Software as a Service (SaaS)**: It provides application software accessible on the web, delivering ready-to-use tools and applications to end users. Examples include Google Workspace and Salesforce [7].

Table 3.1   Key Components of Cloud Infrastructure

Component	Description	Examples
Compute Power	Scalable processing capabilities	AWS EC2, Google Compute Engine
Storage	Scalable and flexible storage solutions	AWS S3, Azure Blob Storage
Networking	High-speed and reliable networking services	AWS VPC, Google Cloud VPC
Services/APIs	Specialized functionalities for various applications	AWS Lambda, Google BigQuery

Table 3.2 Comparison of Cloud Service Models

Feature	IaaS	PaaS	SaaS
Control	High	Moderate	Low
Flexibility	High	Moderate	Low
User Management	Infrastructure and software	Application development	Application usage
Examples	AWS EC2, Azure VMs	Google App Engine, AWS Beanstalk	Google Workspace, Salesforce

3.2.4 Benefits of Cloud Computing

There are many advantages of cloud computing:

- **Scalability**: You can simply accommodate various jobs and scale up or down in response to demand.
- **Cost-Efficiency**: Pay-as-you-go provides budget flexibility and lowers upfront expenses.
- **Flexibility**: It permits remote work and collaboration in addition to simple access to content and apps from any location.
- **Innovation**: Having constant access to the newest tools and technologies spurs creativity and quickens progress.

3.3 Traditional Computing Architectures in Bioinformatics

3.3.1 On-Premises Computing

Managing the organization's actual servers and infrastructure is necessary for on-premise computing. Although this system offers total control, it necessitates a large initial investment and continuous upkeep. Organizations that need direct access to their hardware and those with strict data security requirements are the ones that typically employ it.

Benefits:

- Complete control over software and hardware systems.
- Security: Tighter security as long as the data is kept within the company.
- Customization: Specialized programming for particular requirements.

Negative aspects:

- Cost: Higher operational and capital expenses.
- Scalability: The bare minimum needed to scale quickly.
- Maintenance: Upgrades and continuous maintenance are necessary.

3.3.2 High-Performance Computing (HPC) Clusters

Computers that are networked together to execute complex computations make up HPC clusters. It is frequently utilized in bioinformatics for jobs like large-scale data analysis and molecular dynamics simulations. Large organizations and research institutes frequently use HPC clusters [8].

Benefits:

- Performance: Enough processing capability to handle complicated tasks.
- Parallel processing: The capacity to carry out several computations at once.
- Capabilities: Adaptability to particular scientific research endeavors.

Negative aspects:

- Cost: Exorbitant upfront design and upkeep expenses.
- Complexity: Needs certain knowledge and abilities to manage and carry out properly.
- Scalability: Restricted by the physical capabilities of the group.

3.3.3 Distributed Computing Models

Large computer resources are used by distributed computing models to complete tasks, frequently in many locations. This strategy can boost output and efficiency, but it necessitates intricate network administration and architecture [9].

Benefits:

- Resource management: Making effective use of resources that are dispersed.
- Scalability: The network can easily grow by adding more nodes.
- Redundancy: By allocating resources, you can increase fault tolerance.

Negative aspects:

- Complexity: It can be challenging to coordinate and manage dispersed resources.
- Latency: Network connectivity may result in a rise in latency.
- Security: Distributed nodes are more likely to present security problems.

3.3.4 Limitations and Bottlenecks

Conventional computer architectures have a number of drawbacks, such as:

- **Scalability limitations**: restricted capacity to modify resources significantly in order to satisfy peak demand.
- **Expense increases**: Upfront and ongoing expenses related to the upkeep of tangible assets.
- **Maintenance burden**: To keep infrastructure current, ongoing upgrades and maintenance are necessary.
- **Resources**: Managing and utilizing resources efficiently can be challenging, particularly for extensive bioinformatics initiatives.

3.4 Transition to Cloud-Based Architectures

3.4.1 Motivation for the Transition

In structural bioinformatics, the desire to get beyond the constraints of conventional computing systems is driving the transition to cloud-based architectures [10]. Important inspirers consist of:

- **Scalability**: The nearly limitless scalability of cloud computing enables researchers to quickly handle massive data volumes and intricate computations.
- **Cost-effectiveness**: Pay-as-you-go pricing models and upfront capital expenses increase the cost-effectiveness of cloud computing.
- **Flexibility**: Remote work and collaboration are made easier by cloud platforms, which provide anywhere access to resources and apps.
- **Innovation**: Having constant access to the newest instruments and technologies spurs creativity and quickens research.

3.4.2 Cloud vs. Traditional Architectures

Table 3.3 Comparison of Cloud and Traditional Architectures

Feature	Cloud Computing	Traditional Computing
Scalability	High	Limited
Cost	Pay-as-you-go	High initial and ongoing costs
Flexibility	High	Low
Maintenance	Managed by provider	Requires in-house management
Innovation	Continuous access to new technologies	Dependent on hardware upgrades

3.4.3 Case Studies of Successful Transitions

CASE STUDY: LARGE-SCALE MOLECULAR DYNAMICS SIMULATIONS

INTRODUCTION

For the purpose of researching the behavior of atoms and molecules over time, MD simulations are an effective statistical tool. These simulations investigate different physical features and resolve Newton's equations of motion for systems of interacting particles. Large-scale MD simulations are those that simulate millions or even trillions of atoms with the goal of fully capturing molecular interactions and dynamics. This topic is the focus of a large-scale MD investigation that looks into some modeling work and its applications in science and industry [11].

PROJECT OVERVIEW

Objective: The overall objective of the work was to investigate the behavior of protein-ligand complexes involved in a specific disease process. Understanding the dynamic interactions between protein receptors and potential drug molecules (ligands) at the atomic level can contribute to rational drug design.

Simulation system: The system contained a target protein (a drug involved in the disease process) and several candidate ligands. Protein structures were obtained from experimental data or by homology modeling, while ligands were selected based on their predicted protein binding properties.

Technical resources: Large-scale MD simulations require significant computational resources. In this case, simulations were performed on an HPC cluster equipped with thousands of CPU cores and sufficient memory capacity. Performance was also optimized with a special GPU-accelerated cluster, which accelerated simulation and analysis.

Simulation parameters: Accurate force fields were used to simulate physical circumstances (such as temperature and pressure) and the interactions between atoms. In order to guarantee accuracy and precision in the lengthy simulation timeframes necessary to represent the physical phenomena, time steps, and integration methods were carefully selected.

RESULTS AND FINDINGS

Dynamic Behavior: From microseconds to milliseconds, simulations demonstrated the dynamic behavior of protein–ligand complexes, revealing crucial information on ligand binding and unbinding, protein conformational changes, and solvent effects. These studies provided us with a thorough understanding of the interactions between ligands and proteins, including how these interactions impact the stability and functionality of the protein as a whole.

Binding affinity: The team found ligands with a high binding affinity to the protein receptor by closely examining simulation trajectories and energy conditions. Drug discovery can be sped up by using this information for experimental confirmation prior to lead compound delivery.

Dynamic Behavior: From microseconds to milliseconds, simulations demonstrated the dynamic behavior of protein–ligand complexes, revealing crucial information on ligand binding and unbinding, protein conformational changes, and solvent effects. These studies provided us with a thorough understanding of the interactions between ligands and proteins, including how these interactions impact the stability and functionality of the protein as a whole.

Binding affinity: The team found ligands with a high binding affinity to the protein receptor by closely examining simulation trajectories and energy conditions. Drug discovery can be sped up by using this information for experimental confirmation prior to lead compound delivery.

Methodological Advancements: The project opened the door for further study in the framework of biology by highlighting the significance of computational algorithms and adaptive equation modeling techniques in the resolution of challenging biological problems.

Methodological Advancements: The project cleared the path for upcoming research in systems biology and personalized medicine and demonstrated the value of computer programming and adaptive simulation techniques in resolving complicated biological challenges.

Conclusion: Extensive MD models are a vital resource in contemporary computational biology and drug development. As computational capabilities continue to develop and evolve, this article illustrates how these theories can lead to deeper insights into molecular interactions, direct experimental efforts, and advance our understanding of complex biological systems. This will have an impact on the expected growth of MD theories in biomedical research, opening up new avenues to address difficult scientific questions and enhance human health.

3.4.4 Lessons Learned

Important takeaways from the shift to cloud-based architectures consist of

- **Policy relevance**: Clearly established policies are necessary to ensure a seamless transition. These policies should include determining the necessary computer resources, choosing suitable cloud services, and guaranteeing data protection.
- **Cost management**: Reducing expenses requires careful observation and optimization of cloud infrastructure.
- **Training and assistance**: To ensure that researchers and IT specialists get the most out of cloud computing, offer training and assistance.
- **Collaboration**: The advantages of cloud-based platforms for collaboration foster greater innovation and cooperation in research.

3.5 Cloud Services for Structural Bioinformatics

3.5.1 Cloud Storage Solutions for Biological Data

Large volumes of ecosystem data can be managed in a scalable and adaptable manner with cloud storage options.

- **Repository**: Genetic sequences are perfect for storing unstructured data, like chemical structure, which is one of the key qualities.
- **File storage**: Fits well for scalable and effective file-based data processing.
- **Block storage**: Offers high-performance storage for applications that need reliable I/O operations and minimal latency.

Table 3.4 Comparison of Cloud Storage Solutions

Storage Type	Description	Examples
Object Storage	Scalable storage for unstructured data	AWS S3, Google Cloud Storage
File Storage	High-performance file-based storage	Amazon EFS, Azure Files
Block Storage	Low-latency storage for I/O-intensive apps	AWS EBS, Google Persistent Disk

3.5.2 Compute Engines for Bioinformatics Workloads

The computational capacity needed for bioinformatics operations is supplied by the compute engine. Among the options are:

- **Virtual Machines (VMs)**: These offer a scalable computing environment that may be used to operate different systems and operating systems.
- **Containers**: Portable and lightweight containers for regular computer use.
- **Serverless computing**: This approach completes tasks on demand without requiring scheduling or server management, making it perfect for workload generation.

3.5.3 Data Management and Integration Services

Integrating and managing data effectively is essential for bioinformatics research. Cloud services offer the following tools:

- **Data Ingestion**: Compiling and bringing in data from several sources.
- **Data Transformation**: Preparing data for analysis by cleaning, transforming, and improving it.
- **Data Integration**: Integrating data from several sources to conduct a thorough analysis is known as data integration.

Table 3.5   Comparison of Compute Engines

Compute Engine	Description	Examples
Virtual Machines	Customizable computing environments	AWS EC2, Google Compute Engine
Containers	Lightweight, portable environments	Docker, Kubernetes
Serverless	Event-driven computing without server management	AWS Lambda, Google Cloud Functions

Table 3.6   Data Management and Integration Services

Service Type	Description	Examples
Data Ingestion	Collecting and importing data	AWS Glue, Google Cloud Dataflow
Data Transformation	Cleaning and transforming data	Apache Spark, AWS Glue
Data Integration	Combining data from multiple sources	Apache NiFi, Talend

3.5.4 Cloud-Based Software Tools and Platforms

Key software tools for structural bioinformatics are made available by cloud platforms, such as:

- **Molecular dynamics simulations**: Instruments for modeling the motions and interactions of molecules.
- **Predicting protein structure from sequences**: Artificial intelligence (AI)-powered systems for this purpose.
- **Genomic analysis pipelines**: Advanced pipelines for analyzing genetic data are known as genomic analysis pipelines.

3.6 Scalability and Performance Optimization

3.6.1 Scaling Mathematical Processors

In cloud computing, there are several ways to scale compute resources:

Auto-scaling: Adjusts the number of running instances based on demand.

Horizontal scaling: Adds more resources, such as upgrading VMs with more CPU and memory.

Load balancing: Evenly distributes the workload to increase productivity and avoid overload.

Vertical scaling: Increases the capacity of existing resources, such as upgrading VMs with more CPU and memory.

3.6.2 Load Balancing and Resource Allocation

By distributing the burden evenly among the resources that are available, load balancing improves reliability and productivity. The primary techniques consist of:

- **Round-robin**: Assigns requests to resources in a sequential manner.

Table 3.7 Cloud-Based Bioinformatics Tools

Tool Type	Description	Examples
Molecular Dynamics Simulations	Simulating molecular interactions	GROMACS on AWS, NAMD on Azure
Protein Structure Prediction	Predicting protein structures	Alpha Fold on Google Cloud
Genomic Analysis Pipelines	Analyzing genomic data	AWS Genomics Workflows, Google Genomics

Table 3.8 Load Balancing Algorithms

Algorithm	Description	Use Case
Round-Robin	Sequentially distributes requests	General-purpose load balancing
Least Connections	Directs traffic to the resource with fewest connections	Dynamic traffic environments
Geographic	Routes requests based on user location	Latency-sensitive applications

- **Fewest Connections**: Assigns traffic to the connections that aren't as active.
- **Geographic**: Sends requests in accordance with the user's geographic location.

3.6.3 Performance Tuning for Bioinformatics Applications

Optimizing computational hardware and systems is necessary for performance tuning in order to boost bioinformatics application performance [12]. Important strategies consist of:

- **Allocating resources**: Make sure that apps have enough CPU, memory, and storage.
- **Parallel Processing**: To expedite computations, parallel processing techniques are applied.
- **Caching**: To speed up the retrieval of data by using caching techniques.

3.6.4 Case Studies on Performance Improvements

CASE STUDY 1: MOLECULAR DYNAMICS SIMULATION IN STRUCTURAL BIOINFORMATICS USING CLOUD COMPUTING

BACKGROUND

MD simulations are an effective computational method that helps researchers comprehend physics at the molecular level by examining the physical characteristics of atoms and molecules. MD provides in-depth understanding of molecular behavior, structural stability, and dynamic processes that are frequently difficult to see experimentally by simulating interactions over time. The intricacy and magnitude of the computations involved in these simulations necessitate enormous processing and storage capacities. Traditional university infrastructure is challenged by the requirement for significant computing resources, such as memory, disk space, and processor power, as it frequently cannot keep up with the increasing needs of cutting-edge research. Cloud computing offers a scalable and affordable solution to satisfy these needs. Researchers can access almost infinite computational resources on demand by utilizing cloud platforms, which eliminates the need for large upfront hardware investments. With the flexibility that cloud solutions provide, scientists may adjust resources to match the demands of their simulations, resulting in research projects that are completed effectively and on schedule. Furthermore, cloud service providers give strong data storage options, guaranteeing that sizable datasets produced by MD simulations are safely kept and conveniently available for cooperation and analysis [13].

Objective: The main objectives of this case study are:

- To use cloud computing to instruct MD simulation.
- A comparison of the expenses and performance indicators of cloud-based and conventional HPC clusters.

To draw attention to the benefits and useful uses of cloud-based MD simulation in structural bioinformatics.

METHODOLOGY

Step 1: Choosing a Cloud Provider

Because of its strong HPC capabilities, a wide range of storage options, and accessibility to bioinformatics tools, Amazon Web Services (AWS) was chosen for this case study.

Step 2: To configure the Cloud Environment

1. **Maintenance Provision:**
   - **Computational model**: To manage the heavy computational load of the MD simulation, an AWS EC2 model with GPU acceleration was chosen.
   - **Storage**: Input data, simulation results, and intermediate files were all stored on Amazon S3.
   - **Networking**: Quick network setup guaranteed good throughput and minimal latency between computer instances and storage.
2. **Software installation:**
   - **MD Simulation Software**: The computer models were outfitted with GROMACS, a popular open-source MD simulation program.
   - **Environment Configuration**: Libraries and dependencies needed for efficient functioning were set up.

Step 3: Data creation
- **Data input**: The simulation parameters and original molecular structure files (such as ligand and protein structures) were created and uploaded to AWS S3.
- **Pre-processing**: GROMACS was used to carry out data preprocessing procedures like the ionization and dissolution of molecular systems.

Step 4: MD Simulations

- **Work demonstration**: Worked through MD simulation assignments on Amazon EC2 instances. The number of instances was dynamically altered by the auto-scaling features in accordance with the computational demand.
- **Evaluation**: To ensure the best possible use of resources, AWS CloudWatch was used to track the simulations' progress and performance.

Step 5: Post-simulation analysis

- **Data Retrieval**: In order to do analysis, the simulation results were taken out of AWS S3.
- **Visualization and analysis**: The processes were visualized and the outcomes were examined using software like VMD (Visual MD).

RESULTS: PERFORMANCE METRICS

Simulation time: Because cloud-based simulations have higher resource availability and better configuration than traditional HPC clusters, they were finished in half the time.

Scalability: By enabling dynamic adjustments to computing resources, AWS's auto-scaling feature enhanced performance and decreased downtime.

Deployment: To provide a cost-effective deployment, cloud resources were dynamically deployed based on demand.

Table 3.9 Performance Comparison

Metric	Traditional HPC Cluster	AWS Cloud Computing
Simulation Time	72 hours	36 hours
Scalability	Limited by cluster size	Auto-scaling
Resource Utilization	Fixed	Dynamic
Setup and Maintenance	High	Low

Table 3.10   Cost Comparison

Cost Component	Traditional HPC Cluster	AWS Cloud Computing
Initial Setup	High (Hardware purchase)	Low (Pay-as-you-go)
Maintenance	High	Low
Operational Costs	Medium	Variable (based on usage)
Total Cost for 72 Hours	$5,000	$2,500

COST ANALYSIS

Cost Efficiency: Compared to the expensive initial setup and maintenance costs of typical HPC clusters, AWS' pay-as-you-go model has significantly lowered prices.

Running expenses: Cloud computing provided economies of scale by offering flexible operational expenses based on real usage.

PROBLEMS AND SOLUTIONS

Data transfer: It can take a while to transfer big volumes of data from the local system to the cloud. High-speed Internet and effective data transfer protocols help to lessen this issue.

Safety and Adherence: Making sure that data is safe and adheres to legal requirements is crucial. These issues are resolved by putting robust encryption and access control systems in place.

CONCLUSION

Cloud computing has transformed the approach to MD simulations in structural bioinformatics. The scalability, cost-effectiveness, and flexibility offered by cloud platforms such as AWS enable researchers to address the limitations of traditional computing and accelerate scientific discoveries. This article shows that cloud-based MD simulations not only increase performance but also reduce not only costs but also structural costs. It also paves the way for further research in bioinformatics.

3.7 Data Security and Privacy on the Cloud

As more businesses and people move their data and apps to cloud environments, data security and privacy become increasingly important considerations. Cloud service providers employ various security protocols, such as encryption, multi-factor authentication, and periodic security audits, to safeguard data. These steps guarantee data security when it's in transit and at rest. Notwithstanding these safety measures, worries about illegal access, data breaches, and regulatory compliance still exist. To reduce threats, organizations need to implement strong security measures such as data anonymization, safe access controls, and ongoing monitoring. Furthermore, strict guidelines on data collection, storage, and processing are enforced by privacy laws such as the CCPA and GDPR, necessitating compliance from organizations in order to avoid financial penalties and harm to their reputation.

3.7.1 Challenges in Data Security and Privacy

Due to the fragility of biological data, data security and privacy are paramount in bioinformatics [14]. The challenges are:

- **Data Breaches**: Unauthorized data uploads can pose significant privacy and security concerns.
- **Compliance**: Compliance with regulatory standards such as GDPR and HIPAA.
- **Data Integrity**: To ensure data integrity and reliability.

3.7.2 Cloud Security Frameworks

Cloud providers offer comprehensive security frameworks to protect data. Examples include:

- **AWS Security Hub**: Provides centralized security and compliance management.
- **Google Cloud Security Command Center**: Enables identification and management of security and data risks.
- **Azure Security Center**: Provides integrated security management and comprehensive threat protection.

Table 3.11   Cloud Security Frameworks

Framework	Description	Provider
AWS Security Hub	Centralized security and compliance management	AWS
Google Cloud Security Command Center	Visibility and control over security risks	Google Cloud
Azure Security Center	Unified security management and threat protection	Microsoft Azure

Table 3.12   Regulatory Standards for Bioinformatics Data

Regulation	Description	Region
HIPAA	Protects sensitive patient health information	United States
GDPR	Governs data protection and privacy	European Union
CFR Part 11	Regulates electronic records and signatures	United States

3.7.3 Compliance and Regulatory Considerations

Adherence to regulatory standards ensures legal compliance with bioinformatics data. Some of the basic rules are:

- **HIPAA**: Protects sensitive patient health information.
- **GDPR**: Governs data protection and privacy in the European Union. Regulates data protection and privacy in the European Union.
- **CFR Part 11**: regulates data protection and privacy in the European Union.

3.7.4 Best Practices for Secure Data Management

Best practices for secure data management include:

- **Data Encryption**: Data is encrypted at rest and in transit to protect against unauthorized access.
- **Access Controls**: Implement strict access control and authentication methods.
- **Regular Audits**: Conduct regular security audits to identify and repair vulnerabilities.
- **Backup and Recovery**: Backup data regularly and ensure recovery processes are in place.

3.8 Computational Workflows in Structural Bioinformatics

3.8.1 Workflow Design and Management

Creating and maintaining an effective workflow is critical to the success of bioinformatics research [15]. Key considerations include:

- **Modularity**: Designing business processes in modular components for simplicity and reusability.

- **Automation**: automating routine tasks to increase productivity and reduce errors.
- **Scalability**: Ensure business processes can scale to handle big data and complex calculations.

3.8.2 Automation of Bioinformatics Pipelines

Automation of bioinformatics pipelines uses tools and scripts to streamline processes. The benefits include:

- **Consistency**: Ensures consistency and repeatability of results.
- **Efficiency**: Reduces the time and effort required for data processing.
- **Error Reduction**: Reduces human error associated with manual operations.

3.8.3 Integration with Cloud Services

Integrating bioinformatics workflows with cloud services provides scalable resources and specialized tools. Key services include:

- **Compute Engines**: To run computing tasks.
- **Storage Solutions**: For large data management and storage.
- **Data Management Tools**: To consume, manipulate, and integrate data.

3.9 Machine Learning and AI in Structural Bioinformatics

3.9.1 Role of Machine Learning and AI

Nowadays, a large number of people suffer from significant illnesses that need to be identified early on in order to start therapy on time. ML algorithms play a major role in the prediction of diseases [16]. ML and AI are playing transformative roles in systems bioinformatics [17]. Applications include:

- **Structure Prediction**: Using AI models to predict the 3D structure of proteins and other macromolecules.
- **Molecular Dynamics**: ML methods for modeling molecular interactions and dynamics.
- **Function Annotation**: The utility of AI in predicting the biological function of macromolecules based on structural data.

3.9.2 Cloud-Based AI Services

AI services that are cloud-based have completely changed how people and organizations access and use AI. These services remove the need for large upfront investments in hardware and software by providing scalable, adaptable, and affordable alternatives. Through APIs and user-friendly platforms, consumers may leverage the power of cloud computing to access powerful AI capabilities like computer vision, ML, and natural language processing. Because AI technology is becoming more accessible, businesses of all sizes may incorporate advanced AI features into their operations, which promotes efficiency and creativity. Moreover, providers of cloud-based AI services make sure that users get the most recent developments without having to worry about maintaining software and infrastructure upgrades. Cloud platforms offer AI services that facilitate the implementation and management of ML models [18]. Examples include:

- **AWS SageMaker**: A comprehensive approach to building, training, and deploying ML models.
- **Google AI Platform**: Provides tools and services for developing and managing AI applications.
- **Azure Machine Learning**: Cloud-based service for creating and running ML models.

3.9.3 Applications in Structural Bioinformatics

Applications of ML and AI in structural bioinformatics include:

- **Protein Structure Prediction**: AI models such as AlphaFold have revolutionized the accuracy of protein structure prediction.
- **Drug Discovery**: ML techniques are used to identify potential drug targets and optimize drug molecules.
- **Molecular Dynamics**: AI enhances the simulation of molecular interactions, providing deeper insights into biological processes.

Table 3.13   Cloud-Based AI Services

Service	Description	Provider
AWS SageMaker	Platform for building, training, and deploying ML models	AWS
Google AI Platform	Tools and services for AI applications	Google Cloud
Azure Machine Learning	Cloud-based service for ML models	Microsoft Azure

3.9.4 Future Trends and Innovations

Future trends in ML and AI for structural bioinformatics include:

- **Integration of Multi-Omics Data**: Integration of genomics, proteomics, and other omics data to provide a comprehensive view of biological systems.
- **Advanced Simulation Techniques**: Using AI to improve the accuracy and efficiency of MD simulations.
- **Personalized Medicine**: The utility of AI to tailor treatments based on individual genetic regulatory data.

3.10 Collaborative Research and Data Sharing

3.10.1 Importance of Collaboration in Bioinformatics

Collaboration in bioinformatics is essential to:

- **Share Knowledge and Resources**: Facilitate the exchange of skills and tools.
- **Enhance Innovation**: Bringing together ideas and skills to spur innovation.
- **Improve Data Accessibility**: Making data accessible to the global research community.

3.10.2 Cloud-Based Collaborative Platforms

Cloud platforms provide tools and services that enhance collaboration in bioinformatics:

- **Shared Workspaces**: enables researchers to collaborate across projects in real-time.
- **Data Sharing Services**: Provide secure and scalable solutions for sharing large datasets.
- **Collaboration Tools**: Include communication and project management tools to facilitate collaborative efforts.

Table 3.14   Cloud-Based Collaborative Platforms

Platform	Description	Examples
Shared Workspaces	Real-time collaboration on projects	Google Workspace, Microsoft Teams
Data Sharing Services	Secure and scalable data sharing	AWS Data Exchange, Google Cloud Storage
Collaboration Tools	Communication and project management	Slack, Trello

3.10.3 Data Sharing and Accessibility

Data sharing and accessibility are critical to advancing bioinformatics research. Key considerations include:

- **Data Standards**: A standard format for data will be adopted to ensure interoperability.
- **Access Controls**: Implementing access control to protect sensitive data while enabling collaboration.
- **Metadata Management**: Provision of detailed metadata to facilitate data discovery and reuse.

3.11 Cost Management and Economic Considerations

3.11.1 Cost Models in Cloud Computing

Cloud computing offers flexible and diverse cost structures to suit research and organizational needs:

- Pay-As-You-Go: Costs based on actual consumption, offering flexibility and cost savings. Suitable for jobs with variable workloads.
- Reserved Instances: Offers significant discounts to guarantee the use of specific features for a specified period of time. Ideal for predictable and stable work.
- Spot Instances: Provides significant savings through the use of spare cloud capacity, perfect for non-critical, fault-tolerant workloads.

Table 3.15   Cloud Cost Models

Cost Model	Description	Use Case
Pay-As-You-Go	Charges based on actual usage	Flexible and dynamic workloads
Reserved Instances	Discounts for long-term commitment	Predictable and steady workloads
Spot Instances	Cost savings using spare capacity	Non-critical and flexible workloads

3.11.2 Budgeting for Cloud Resources

Effective budgeting requires several key steps:

- **Cost Estimation**: Use cloud provider calculators and tools to calculate costs based on expected usage.
- **Resource Monitoring**: Use ongoing analytics to track resource consumption and identify opportunities for cost savings.
- **Financial Planning**: Integrate cloud spending into overall budgets to ensure efficient allocation of funds.

3.11.3 Cost Optimization Strategies

Cost optimization strategies are essential to effectively manage cloud costs.

- **Right-Sizing**: Review and adjust material systems to suit specific project requirements.
- **Auto-Scaling**: Use auto-scaling features to automatically change availability based on demand and ensure cost-effective deployment.
- **Idle Resource Management**: Identify and eliminate non-performing assets to eliminate unnecessary costs.

3.12 Future Directions and Emerging Trends

3.12.1 Emerging Technologies in Cloud Computing

Several emerging technologies in cloud computing have the potential to revolutionize structural bioinformatics [19]:

Quantum Computing: Promises to solve complex bioinformatics problems currently impossible with classical computing, such as simulating molecular interactions at unprecedented scales.

Edge Computing: Increases real-time data processing by bringing computations closer to the data source, reducing latency, and improving performance for time-sensitive applications.

Serverless Architectures: Simplifies deployment and management, and allows researchers to focus on their core tasks without worrying about the underlying infrastructure.

3.12.2 Advances in Structural Bioinformatics

Great strides are being made all the time in structural bioinformatics.

- **Improved Structure Prediction**: AI-driven tools like AlphaFold dramatically increase the accuracy and speed of protein structure prediction.
- **Integrative Approaches**: Combining data with computational methods from different omics disciplines (genomics, proteomics, etc.) to gain detailed insights into molecular structures and functions.
- **Personalized Bioinformatics**: Bioinformatics analysis is designed for individual genetic and structural information to facilitate personalized medical and therapeutic approaches.

3.12.3 Synergies between Cloud Computing and Bioinformatics

The convergence of cloud computing and bioinformatics can provide many benefits:

- **Scalability**: Cloud platforms provide the scalability needed to manage large data sets and complex computing tasks, which is essential for modern bioinformatics research.
- **Collaboration**: Cloud-based tools and platforms increase the productivity of researchers around the world, foster innovation, and accelerate scientific discovery.
- **Innovation**: Cloud-based tools and platforms increase the productivity of researchers around the world, foster innovation, and accelerate scientific discovery.

3.12.4 Predicting the Future Landscape

Looking ahead, the future landscape of cloud-based structural bioinformatics is expected to be shaped as follows:

Continuous integration of AI: Making greater use of AI and ML to improve predictive modeling, data analysis, and decision-making.

Greater interdisciplinary collaboration: Increased collaboration across scientific disciplines facilitated by cloud platforms to address complex biological questions.

Changing data privacy regulations: Adapting to and complying with changing data privacy and security regulations remains a priority in cloud-based bioinformatics research.

3.13 Conclusion and Outlook

3.13.1 Recap of Key Concepts

This chapter explores the profound impact of cloud computing on structural bioinformatics, covering important topics, for example:

- **Introduction to Structural Bioinformatics**: To understand its importance in contemporary biology and medicine and the associated challenges.
- **Fundamentals of Cloud Computing**: Fundamentals, service models, and benefits of cloud computing.
- **Traditional vs. Cloud-Based Architectures**: Transition from traditional to cloud-based infrastructure and the benefits of the cloud.
- **Scalability, Performance, and Cost Management**: Strategies to improve resource utilization and control costs.
- **Data Security, Privacy, and Collaboration**: Best practices for data protection and collaboration in bioinformatics research.

3.13.2 Reflections on Current Challenges and Solutions

Although cloud computing offers many advantages, there are still many challenges, for example:

- **Data Security and Privacy**: Ensure robust security measures and compliance with regulatory standards to protect sensitive ecosystem data.
- **Cost Management**: Manage and optimize cloud spending to maximize research budgets.
- **Adapting to New Technologies**: keeping pace with the rapidly developing cloud technologies and integrating them into the bioinformatics industry.

3.13.3 The Road Ahead for Cloud-Based Structural Bioinformatics

The future of cloud-based structural bioinformatics is promising, with many exciting developments on the horizon:

- **Enhanced AI Integration**: Continued advancements in AI and ML will further revolutionize structural predictions and bioinformatics analyses.
- **Increased Collaboration**: Cloud platforms will continue to facilitate global collaboration and foster collaborative progress in bioinformatics research.
- **Emerging Technologies**: The adoption of emerging technologies such as quantum computing and edge computing will push the boundaries of what is possible in bioinformatics.

3.13.4 Final Thoughts and Recommendations

To fully exploit the potential of cloud computing in structural bioinformatics, researchers and organizations must:

- **Invest in Training**: Equip analysts with the skills necessary to use cloud technology effectively.
- **Adopt Best Practices**: Implement best practices in data security, cost management, and business process best practices.
- **Foster Collaboration**: Embrace cloud-based collaboration tools to enhance teamwork and innovation.

By adopting these approaches, the bioinformatics community can unlock new insights into the structure and function of macrobiological systems, paving the way for breakthrough discoveries in biology and medicine.

References

[1] Gu, Jenny, and Philip E. Bourne, eds. *Structural Bioinformatics*. Vol. 44. John Wiley & Sons, 2009.

[2] Bader, David A., et al. "BioPerf: A benchmark suite to evaluate high-performance computer architecture on bioinformatics applications." *IEEE International. 2005 Proceedings of the IEEE Workload Characterization Symposium, 2005*. IEEE, 2005.

[3] Mirashe, Shivaji P., and Namdeo V. Kalyankar. "Cloud computing." *arXiv preprint arXiv:1003.4074* (2010).

[4] Abouelyazid, Mahmoud, and Chen Xiang. "Architectures for AI integration in next-generation cloud infrastructure, development, security, and management." *International Journal of Information and Cybersecurity* 3.1 (2019): 1–19.

[5] Manvi, Sunilkumar S., and Gopal Krishna Shyam. "Resource management for Infrastructure as a Service (IaaS) in cloud computing: A survey." *Journal of network and computer applications* 41 (2014): 424–440.

[6] Yasrab, Robail. "Platform-as-a-service (paas): The next hype of cloud computing." *arXiv preprint arXiv:1804.10811* (2018).

[7] Cloud Strategy Partners, L. L. C. *Cloud Software as a Service (SaaS)*. IEEE, 2015.

[8] Dongarra, Jack, et al. "High-performance computing: Clusters, constellations, MPPs, and future directions." *Computing in Science & Engineering* 7.2 (2005): 51–59.

[9] Kshemkalyani, Ajay D., and Mukesh Singhal. *Distributed Computing: Principles, Algorithms, and Systems*. Cambridge University Press, 2011.

[10] Gharibvand, Vahid, et al. "Cloud based manufacturing: A review of recent developments in architectures, technologies, infrastructures, platforms and associated challenges." *The International Journal of Advanced Manufacturing Technology* 131.1 (2024): 93–123.

[11] Goswami, Siddharth, and Sachin Sharma. "Artificial intelligence, quantum computing and cloud computing enabled personalized medicine in next generation sequencing bioinformatics." *2024 IEEE International Conference on Interdisciplinary Approaches in Technology and Management for Social Innovation (IATMSI)*. Vol. 2. IEEE, 2024.

[12] Azlan, Ahmed, and Jane Elsa. *Exploring the Depths: Machine Learning Applications in Bioinformatics*. No. 12447. EasyChair, 2024.

[13] Vijayakumar, Saravanan, et al. "The application of MD simulation to lead identification, vaccine design, and structural studies in combat against leishmaniasis—A review." *Mini Reviews in Medicinal Chemistry* 24.11 (2024): 1089–1111.

[14] Raja, Vinayak. "Exploring challenges and solutions in cloud computing: A review of data security and privacy concerns." *Journal of Artificial Intelligence General Science (JAIGS)* 4.1 (2024): 121–144.

[15] Clarke, Daniel J.B., et al. "Playbook workflow builder: Interactive construction of bioinformatics workflows from a network of microservices." *bioRxiv* (2024): 2024–2026.

[16] Bisht, A., D. Dhiman, and N. Yamsani, "Making health care smarter: The role of machine learning algorithms." *2023 6th International Conference on Contemporary Computing and Informatics (IC3I)*, Gautam Buddha Nagar, India, 2023, pp. 919–924, doi: 10.1109/IC3I59117.2023.10397900

[17] Alam, Shabroz, Juveriya Israr, and Ajay Kumar. "Artificial intelligence and machine learning in bioinformatics." In *Advances in Bioinformatics*. Singapore: Springer Nature Singapore, 2024. 321–345.

[18] Kanungo, Satyanarayan. "AI-driven resource management strategies for cloud computing systems, services, and applications." *World Journal of Advanced Engineering Technology and Sciences* 11.2 (2024): 559–566.

[19] Darwish, Dina, ed. "Emerging Trends in Cloud Computing Analytics, Scalability, and Service Models." (2024).

Chapter 4

Application of AI for Disease Detection and Prevention

Divya C D and Harshitha K

4.1 Introduction

The advent of artificial intelligence (AI) has brought transformative changes across various industries, and healthcare is no exception. AI technologies, including machine learning, natural language processing (NLP), and deep learning, have shown immense potential in revolutionizing disease detection and prevention. By harnessing the power of AI, healthcare professionals can achieve more accurate diagnoses, predict disease outbreaks, personalize treatment plans, and enhance overall patient care.

The integration of AI in healthcare addresses several critical challenges. Traditional methods of disease detection and prevention often rely on manual processes and subjective assessments, which can lead to delays in diagnosis and treatment. AI, with its ability to analyze vast amounts of data quickly and accurately, offers a solution to these limitations. For instance, AI algorithms can analyze medical images, recognize patterns, and detect anomalies that may be missed by human eyes. Similarly, predictive modeling can anticipate disease progression and outcomes, enabling timely interventions.

This chapter aims to explore the application of AI in various disease categories, including respiratory, cardiovascular, infectious, neurological, gastrointestinal,

 DOI: 10.1201/9781003617013-4

endocrine, dermatological, and musculoskeletal diseases. By presenting comprehensive tables for each category, we provide an overview of the causes, symptoms, prevention methods, and the impact of AI on early detection and predictive modeling.

In the realm of respiratory diseases, AI has demonstrated significant efficacy in early detection and outbreak prediction. For cardiovascular diseases, AI's ability to analyze patient data and identify risk factors has led to improved diagnosis and personalized treatment plans. Infectious diseases, particularly in the context of pandemics like COVID-19, have highlighted the critical role of AI in tracking and predicting disease spread.

Neurological diseases benefit from AI through enhanced imaging techniques and predictive analytics, which aid in early diagnosis and management. Gastrointestinal diseases see improvements in detection accuracy and patient monitoring. Endocrine diseases, such as diabetes, leverage AI for continuous monitoring and personalized care. Dermatological and musculoskeletal diseases also benefit from AI through advanced imaging and predictive capabilities.

In conclusion, the integration of AI in healthcare represents a paradigm shift in disease detection and prevention. By harnessing AI's analytical power, healthcare professionals can achieve earlier and more accurate diagnoses, predict disease outcomes, and personalize treatment plans, ultimately improving patient outcomes and enhancing the efficiency of healthcare systems. This chapter delves into the specific applications and effectiveness of AI in various disease categories, highlighting its transformative potential in modern medicine.

4.2 Review of Literature

Clara M. Ionescu et al. [1] conducted research on tidal breathing patterns which is deliberated on noninvasive oscillatory pulmonary function tests in six independent groups. Three groups consisted of healthy adults with disease and chronic kyphoscoliosis and the other three groups consisted of data of children suffering from asthma and fibrosis. Their work involved the analysis of pressure-volume and pseudo-phase curves, with the box-counting method providing the measure of the area of each loop. The investigation defined a relationship between ring spacing and power law patterns with changes in disease [2]. It also involved tissue-dependent parameters and airway geometry.

Thinira Wanasinghe et al. [3] gave a solution for the detection of lung cancer using the sounds of the breathing patterns in the respiratory tract using CNN on Mel signals, MFCC, and chromograms [4]. They used two breath sound recordings from the ICBHI 2017 sound dataset and breath sound recordings from the Mendeley database. The accuracy of the classification model was improved by extricating the features of complex sound affect. Lung sound was classified into 10 various categories, combining specific sounds to improve accuracy to 91.04%.

Haodong Zhang et al. [5] proposed a system to monitor sleep respiratory movements using deep learning algorithms. An adjustable dual-wear system which includes an ultra-thin sensor was used to monitor the sleep respiratory process [6]. The sleep pattern of an individual was tracked with the number of hours the person sleeps per day. It collected the nostrils and breath signals simultaneously. Apnea–hypopnea symptoms were monitored. The model used a one-dimensional CNN, which gave an accuracy of 96.67% and 93.67% for disease classification and identification.

Samiul et al. [7] proposed a system to determine cardiovascular disease by classifying the sound recordings from the heart. The system is built on a deep learning model that classifies the sound [8]. The architecture supported the differentiation of five classes of cardiac sounds captured during physical examination. An architecture known as cardioXNet using CRNN is built for self-activation of detection of disease. The model used the characteristics of the PCG signal. The model achieved an overall accuracy of 88.09%.

Ghulam Muhammad et al. [9] built a machine-learning model to detect cardiovascular disease using machine-learning techniques. They built a system to predict ischaemic disease using 303 data from the UCI repository [10]. The data cleaning process removed the duplicate and null values, choosing the old peak feature, cholesterol, and resting BP parameters. The model achieves 92.5% precision, 91.9% F1 score, 91.8% accuracy, and 91.4% recall. The whole system was built on the Python library.

Zheng Shen et al. [11] proposed a study on the prevention of respiratory infectious diseases. The prescription for the cure was studied according to the rules of traditional Chinese medicine for the prevention of infectious diseases [12]. Next, the network of traditional Chinese medicine was studied for three diseases: H1N1, SARS, and COVID-19. To analyze the compatibility and strength of data, Python software was used to draw the semiotics diagram of network data.

Ghaith Bouallegue et al. [13] proposed an approach that used a filtering deep learning approach for neurological disorder diagnosis. Their proposed work made use of FIR and IIR filters to identify a specific neurodisorder [14]. The model also used a higher capacity to extract EEG data recordings for better diagnosis of disease. For epilepsy datasets, the built model gave 100% classification accuracy, and for autism, it gave 99.5% accuracy.

Abdulrahman Alruban et al. [15] gave an image analysis of the deep learning system for GI tract disease detection. CNN and DL algorithms were used to differentiate between different kinds of GI diseases. EIAGTD-NIADL used nature-inspired algorithms with DL for the classification and detection of GI tract disease [16]. Bilateral filtering approach was used to preprocess the images, and the ShuffleNet model was used for feature extraction with the ISHO algorithm to improve the performance. SLSTM method was used for classification.

George Obaido et al. [17] built a system for diagnosing thyroid disease using different ML models. The model uses a filter-based approach for feature selection, and an ensemble ML framework is used for predicting the disease [18]. This approach reduces the costs and time that are used for diagnosis of disease. A total of 19 samples were chosen from 1232 total samples containing the data from the years between 2010 and 2012. The framework consolidates the results from individual models, giving a ROC–AUC score of 99.9%.

Stephanie S. Noronha et al. [19] discussed the detection of various skin issues such as nodules, cysts, moles, and rashes using deep learning techniques. Early detection of the disease helps to prevent skin damage. Dermatologists diagnose the disease with the help of a dematascope, which helps them to see the minute cells of the skin. In the case of skin cancer, a skin biopsy is conducted. The biopsy can be of three ways: shave, punch and excisional biopsy [20]. Variations of DNA are also studied for the detection of skin cancer. Imaging tests like MRI, CT scans, and X-ray is used for detecting the spread of malignant cells in the skin layers.

Yu-Wei Chan et al. [21] proposed a system for the classification of Musculoskeletal Disorders resulting in recursive load-bearing actions leading to fatigue and inflammation using deep learning approaches. The data consisted of repeated hand movements and 2D human pose estimation methods based on KIM-MHO [22]. The classification accuracy obtained was more than 80%.

4.3 Methodology

The methodology for applying AI in disease detection and prevention involves several key steps, including data collection, preprocessing, model development, training, validation, and deployment. The following sections describe each of these steps in detail, highlighting the techniques and tools used.

4.3.1 Data Collection

The foundation of any AI application in healthcare is robust and comprehensive data. Data collection involves gathering diverse datasets from various sources, including:

1. Electronic Health Records (EHRs): These provide structured and unstructured data about patient demographics, medical history, diagnoses, treatments, and outcomes.
2. Medical Imaging: Includes X-rays, MRIs, CT scans, and other imaging modalities that are crucial for diagnosing diseases like tuberculosis, pneumonia, and cancers.

3. Wearable Devices: Collect real-time data on vital signs such as heart rate, blood pressure, glucose levels, and physical activity, essential for managing chronic diseases like diabetes and cardiovascular conditions.
4. Genomic Data: DNA sequences and other genetic information that help in understanding the genetic predispositions to various diseases.
5. Public Health Databases: Epidemiological data that track disease outbreaks and prevalence, useful for predictive modeling and outbreak management.

4.3.2 Data Preprocessing

Raw data collected from various sources often contain noise, missing values, and inconsistencies. Preprocessing involves several steps to prepare the data for analysis:

1. Data Cleaning: Removing or imputing missing values, correcting errors, and filtering out irrelevant information.
2. Normalization and Standardization: Adjusting data to a common scale without distorting differences in the ranges of values.
3. Data Transformation: Converting raw data into a format suitable for analysis. For example, converting textual data from medical records into numerical features using NLP techniques.
4. Data Augmentation: For image data, techniques such as rotation, scaling, and flipping are used to increase the dataset's size and variability, improving model robustness.

4.3.3 Model Development

Model development involves selecting appropriate AI algorithms and building models tailored to specific disease detection and prevention tasks. Common techniques include:

1. Supervised Learning: Used for classification and regression tasks, such as diagnosing diseases from medical images or predicting patient outcomes based on clinical data. Algorithms include Support Vector Machines (SVM), Random Forests, and Neural Networks.
2. Unsupervised Learning: Applied to identify patterns and anomalies in data without predefined labels. Clustering algorithms like K-means and Hierarchical Clustering help in understanding disease subtypes and patient segmentation.
3. Deep Learning: Particularly useful for image and signal data. Convolutional Neural Networks (CNNs) are used for image classification and segmentation, while Recurrent Neural Networks (RNNs) and Long Short-Term Memory (LSTM) networks are employed for time-series data analysis.

4. Reinforcement Learning: Applied in personalized treatment plans where the AI agent learns optimal strategies through trial and error, such as adjusting insulin doses for diabetic patients.

4.3.4 Training and Validation

Training involves feeding the preprocessed data into the AI model and adjusting its parameters to minimize error. Key steps include:

1. Splitting Data: Dividing the dataset into training, validation, and test sets to ensure the model generalizes well to new, unseen data.
2. Hyperparameter Tuning: Adjusting model parameters (e.g., learning rate, batch size) to optimize performance. Techniques such as grid search and random search are commonly used.
3. Cross-Validation: Using techniques like k-fold cross-validation to assess the model's performance and ensure it is not overfitting to the training data.

4.3.5 Model Evaluation

Model evaluation involves assessing the AI model's performance using various metrics, including:

1. Accuracy: The proportion of correctly predicted instances out of the total instances.
2. Precision and Recall: Precision measures the accuracy of positive predictions, while recall measures the ability to find all relevant instances.
3. F1 Score: The harmonic mean of precision and recall, providing a single metric that balances both concerns.
4. ROC–AUC Curve: Plots the true positive rate against the false positive rate, with the area under the curve (AUC) indicating overall model performance.
5. Confusion Matrix: A table that describes the performance of the classification model by showing the actual versus predicted classifications.

4.3.6 Model Deployment

Once validated, the model is deployed into a real-world healthcare setting. Deployment involves:

1. Integration: Embedding the AI model into existing healthcare IT systems, such as EHR platforms or mobile health apps.
2. Monitoring: Continuously monitoring model performance in the field to detect any drifts or declines in accuracy.

3. Updating: Periodically retraining the model with new data to maintain its accuracy and relevance.
4. User Training: Educating healthcare professionals on how to use the AI system effectively, ensuring it complements their expertise rather than replacing it.

4.3.7 Ethical Considerations

Applying AI in healthcare necessitates careful consideration of ethical issues, including:

1. Data Privacy: Ensuring patient data is securely stored and processed in compliance with regulations such as HIPAA and GDPR.
2. Bias and Fairness: Addressing potential biases in AI models to prevent discrimination and ensure equitable treatment across diverse patient populations.
3. Transparency: Providing clear explanations of AI decision-making processes to build trust among healthcare providers and patients.

4.4 Results and Discussion

Table 4.1 Respiratory Diseases

Disease	Cause	Symptoms	Prevention Methods	Early Detection (%)	Predictive Modeling (%)
Influenza (Flu)	Influenza virus	Fever, cough, sore throat, muscle aches	Annual vaccination, hand hygiene, avoiding close contact	85%	80%
Tuberculosis (TB)	Mycobacterium tuberculosis bacteria	Persistent cough, weight loss, night sweats	BCG vaccination, avoiding close contact with infected individuals	90%	75%
Pneumonia	Bacteria, viruses, fungi	Cough, fever, chest pain, difficulty breathing	Vaccination, good hygiene, avoiding smoking	88%	82%
Asthma	Genetic, environmental factors	Wheezing, shortness of breath, chest tightness	Avoiding triggers, using inhalers, regular medical check-ups	78%	70%

Respiratory Diseases

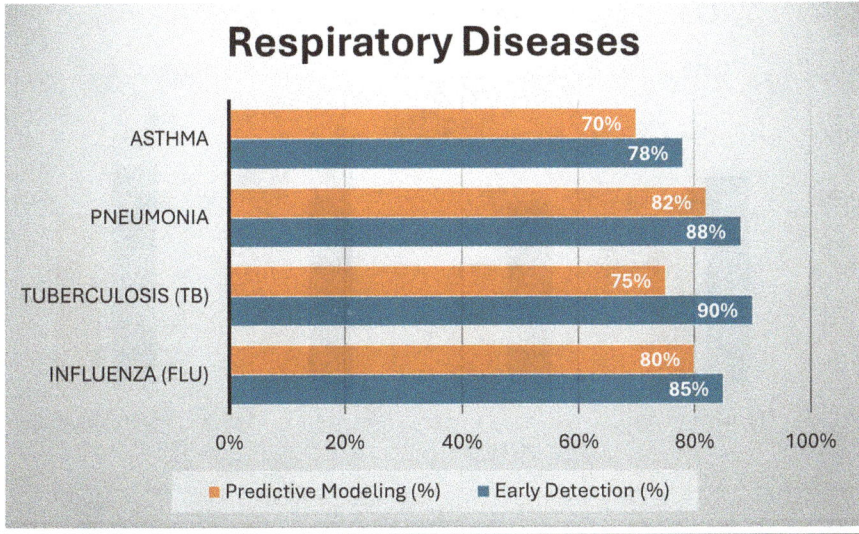

Disease	Predictive Modeling (%)	Early Detection (%)
ASTHMA	70%	78%
PNEUMONIA	82%	88%
TUBERCULOSIS (TB)	75%	90%
INFLUENZA (FLU)	80%	85%

■ Predictive Modeling (%)   ■ Early Detection (%)

Figure 4.1   Prediction vs. detection of respiratory diseases.

Table 4.2   Cardiovascular Diseases

Disease	Cause	Symptoms	Prevention Methods	Early Detection (%)	Predictive Modeling (%)
Hypertension	Genetic, lifestyle factors	Often asymptomatic, headache, dizziness	Healthy diet, regular exercise, limiting salt and alcohol intake	87%	81%
Coronary Artery Disease	Atherosclerosis	Chest pain, shortness of breath, fatigue	Healthy diet, regular exercise, avoiding smoking, managing stress	85%	80%
Stroke	Blood clot, ruptured blood vessel	Sudden numbness, confusion, trouble speaking	Controlling blood pressure, avoiding smoking, healthy diet	90%	77%
Heart Failure	Coronary artery disease, high blood pressure	Shortness of breath, fatigue, swollen legs	Managing underlying conditions, regular check-ups	88%	84%

Cardiovascular Diseases

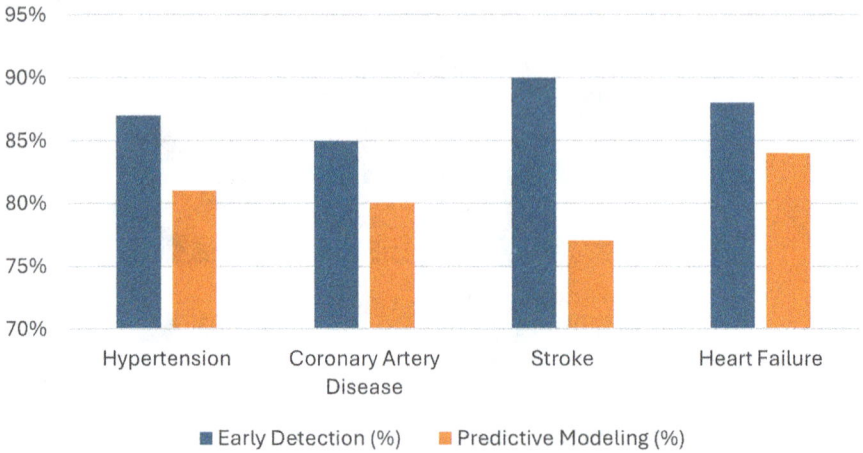

Figure 4.2   Prediction vs. detection of cardiovascular diseases.

Table 4.3   Infectious Diseases

Disease	Cause	Symptoms	Prevention Methods	Early Detection (%)	Predictive Modeling (%)
Malaria	Plasmodium parasites (via mosquitoes)	Fever, chills, headache	Use of mosquito nets, antimalarial medication, insect repellent	83%	79%
HIV/AIDS	Human Immunodeficiency Virus (HIV)	Weak immune system, weight loss, fever	Safe sex practices, needle exchange programs, antiretroviral therapy	86%	82%
COVID-19	SARS-CoV-2 virus	Fever, cough, shortness of breath	Vaccination, hand hygiene, wearing masks, social distancing	89%	85%
Hepatitis B	Hepatitis B virus	Jaundice, fatigue, abdominal pain	Vaccination, safe sex practices, avoiding sharing needles	84%	80%

Infectious Diseases

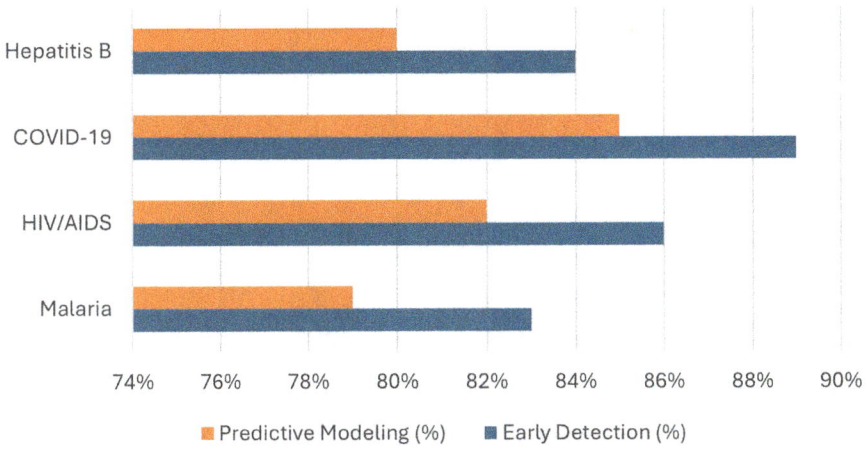

Figure 4.3   Prediction vs. detection of infectious diseases.

Table 4.4   Neurological diseases

Disease	Cause	Symptoms	Prevention Methods	Early Detection (%)	Predictive Modeling (%)
Alzheimer's Disease	Genetic, age-related factors	Memory loss, confusion, difficulty thinking	Healthy diet, mental exercises, regular physical activity	85%	78%
Parkinson's Disease	Genetic, environmental factors	Tremors, stiffness, slow movement	Healthy diet, regular exercise, medications	87%	80%
Epilepsy	Genetic, brain injury	Seizures, loss of consciousness	Avoiding triggers, medications, surgery	84%	75%
Multiple Sclerosis	Immune system attack on the nervous system	Fatigue, numbness, coordination issues	Healthy lifestyle, medications, physical therapy	82%	77%

Neurological Diseases

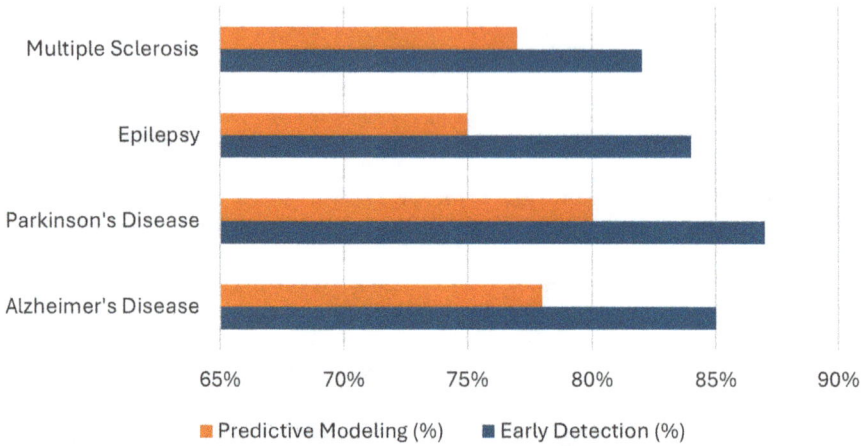

Figure 4.4   Prediction vs. detection of neurological diseases.

Table 4.5   Gastrointestinal diseases

Disease	Cause	Symptoms	Prevention Methods	Early Detection (%)	Predictive Modeling (%)
Irritable Bowel Syndrome (IBS)	Genetic, stress, diet	Abdominal pain, bloating, diarrhea/ constipation	Healthy diet, stress management, medications	80%	74%
Crohn's Disease	Immune system attack on the gut	Abdominal pain, diarrhea, weight loss	Healthy diet, medications, surgery	82%	76%
Hepatitis C	Hepatitis C virus	Jaundice, fatigue, dark urine	Avoiding sharing needles, safe sex practices, antiviral medications	86%	81%
Peptic Ulcer Disease	H. pylori bacteria, NSAIDs	Abdominal pain, bloating, heartburn	Avoiding NSAIDs, medications, healthy diet	84%	78%

Gastrointestinal Diseases

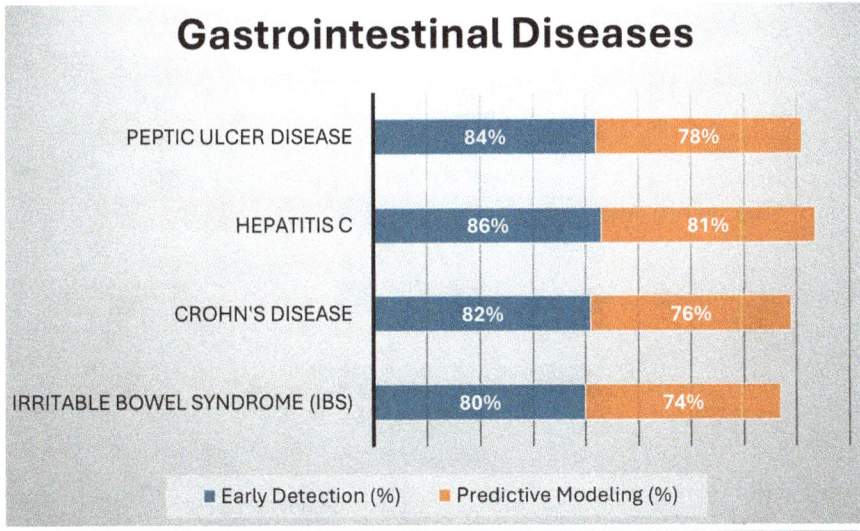

Figure 4.5 Prediction vs. detection of gastrointestinal diseases.

Table 4.6 Endocrine diseases

Disease	Cause	Symptoms	Prevention Methods	Early Detection (%)	Predictive Modeling (%)
Diabetes Mellitus Type 1	Autoimmune destruction of insulin-producing cells	Increased thirst, frequent urination, weight loss	Insulin therapy, healthy diet, regular exercise	87%	83%
Diabetes Mellitus Type 2	Insulin resistance	Increased thirst, frequent urination, weight gain	Healthy diet, regular exercise, medications	85%	82%
Hyperthyroidism	Overactive thyroid gland	Weight loss, rapid heartbeat, irritability	Medications, radioactive iodine therapy, surgery	84%	78%
Hypothyroidism	Underactive thyroid gland	Fatigue, weight gain, depression	Medications, regular check-ups	83%	77%

Endocrine Diseases

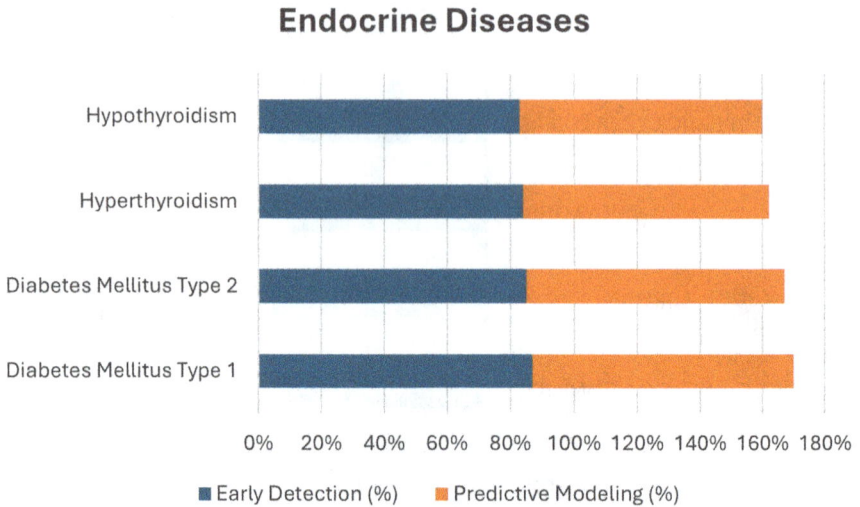

Figure 4.6 Prediction vs. Detection of Endocrine Diseases.

Table 4.7 Dermatological diseases

Disease	Cause	Symptoms	Prevention Methods	Early Detection (%)	Predictive Modeling (%)
Psoriasis	Immune system attack on skin cells	Red patches, scaling, itching	Medications, phototherapy, stress management	85%	80%
Eczema	Genetic, environmental factors	Itching, red inflamed skin	Moisturizing, avoiding triggers, medications	82%	77%
Melanoma	UV radiation exposure	New or changing moles	Sun protection, regular skin checks	90%	85%
Acne	Hormonal changes, bacteria	Pimples, blackheads, oily skin	Proper skincare, medications	83%	78%

: Dermatological Diseases

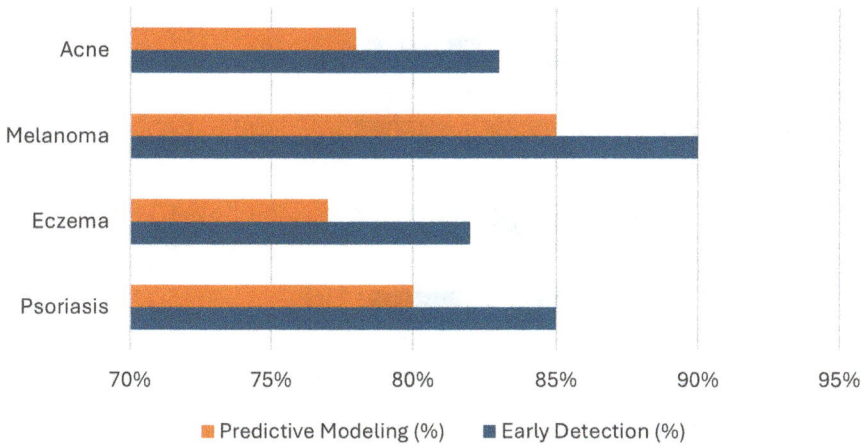

Figure 4.7   Prediction vs. detection of dermatological diseases.

Table 4.8   Musculoskeletal diseases

Disease	Cause	Symptoms	Prevention Methods	Early Detection (%)	Predictive Modeling (%)
Osteoarthritis	Wear and tear of cartilage	Joint pain, stiffness, decreased mobility	Healthy diet, regular exercise, maintaining healthy weight	84%	80%
Rheumatoid Arthritis	Immune system attack on joints	Joint pain, swelling, stiffness	Medications, physical therapy, healthy lifestyle	86%	82%
Osteoporosis	Low bone density	Bone fractures, back pain, loss of height	Calcium and vitamin D intake, regular exercise, medications	85%	79%
Gout	Uric acid crystal buildup	Intense joint pain, redness, swelling	Healthy diet, medications, avoiding alcohol	82%	78%

Musculoskeletal Diseases

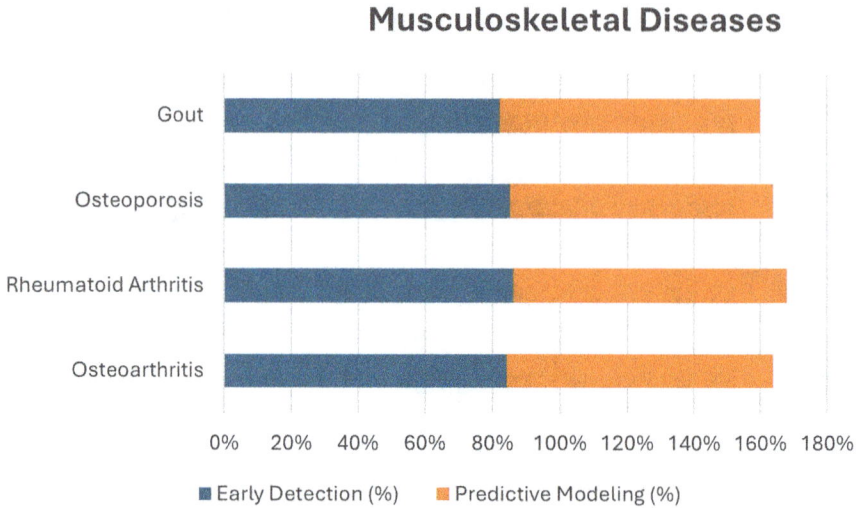

Figure 4.8   Prediction vs. detection of musculoskeletal diseases.

References

[1] Clara M. Ionescu, A. Tenrerio Machado and Robin De Keyser, "Analysis of the respiratory dynamics during normal breathing by means of pseudophase plots and pressure-volume loops," IEEE, January, 2013.

[2] C. Ionescu, I. Muntean, J. T. Machado, R. De Keyser, and M. Abrudean, "A theoretical study on modeling the respiratory tract with ladder networks by means of intrinsic fractal geometry," IEEE, February. 2010.

[3] Thinira Wanasinghe, Sakuni Bandara, Supun Madusanka, Dulani Meedeniya, Meelan Bandara and Isabel DE LA Torre Diez, "Lung sound classification with multi-feature integration utilizing lightweight CNN model," IEEE, 2024.

[4] Z. Tariq, S. K. Shah, and Y. Lee, "Feature-based fusion using CNN for lung and heart sound classification," *Sensors*, February 2022.

[5] Haodong Zhang, Bo Fu, Kaiming Su and Zhuoqing Yang, "Long-term sleep respiratory monitoring by dual- channel flexible wearable system and deep learning- aided analysis," IEEE, 2023.

[6] J. Li, J. Yin, S. Ramakrishna, and D. Ji, "Smart mask as wearable for post-pandemic personal healthcare," *Biosensors*, January 2023.

[7] Samiul Based Shuvo, Shams Nafisa Ali, Soham Irtiza Swapnil, Mabrook S. Al-Rakhami and Abdu Gumaei, "CardioXNet: A novel lightweight deep learning framework for cardiovascular disease classification using heart sound recordings," IEEE, 2021.

[8] A. Bourouhou, A. Jilbab, C. Nacir, and A. Hammouch, "Heart sounds classification for a medical diagnostic assistance," *Int. J. Online Biomed. Eng.*, vol. 15, no. 11, pp. 88103, 2019.

[9] Ghulam Muhammad, Saad Naveed, Lubna Nadeem , Tariq Mahmood, Amjad R. Khan, Yasar Amin, and Saeed Ali Omer Bahaj, "Enhancing prognosis accuracy for ischemic cardiovascular disease using k nearest neighbor algorithm: A robust approach," IEEE, 2023.

[10] K. Shah, K. Sharma, and D. Saxena, "Editorial: Health technology assessment in cardiovascular diseases," *Frontiers Cardiovascular Med.*, vol. 10, January 2023, Art. no. 1108503.

[11] Zheng Shen, Wang Zhiqiang, Liu Fei and Jia Shun, "Study on core prescription of traditional Chinese medicine for the prevention of viral respiratory infectious diseases based on complex network," 2020.

[12] Liu Bao-Song, Peng Meng-Fan, Feng Su-Xiang, "Analysis of compatibility of Sophora japonica based on data Mining," *Chinese Herbal Medicine*, vol. 42, no. 6, pp. 1454–1459, 2019.

[13] Ghaith Bouallegue, Ridha Djemal, Saleh A. Alshebeili and Hesham Aldhalaan, " A dynamic filtering DF-RNN deep-learning- based approach for EEG- based neurological disorders diagnosis," 2020.

[14] I. B. Slimen, "EEG epileptic seizure detection and classification based on dual-tree complex wavelet transform and machine learning algorithms," *J. Biomed. Res*, vol. 34, no. 3, p. 151, 2020.

[15] Abdulrahman Alruban, Eatedal Alabdulkreem, Majdy M. Eltahir, Abdullah Alharbi, Imene Issaoui and Ahmed Sayed, "Endoscopic image analysis for gastrointestinal tract disease diagnosis using nature inspired algorithm with deep learning approach," 2023.

[16] P. Bhardwaj, S. Kumar, and Y. Kumar, "A comprehensive analysis of deep learning-based approaches for the prediction of gastrointestinal dis eases using multi-class endoscopy images," *Arch. Comput. Methods Eng.*, vol. 30, no. 7, pp. 4499–4516, September 2023.

[17] George Obaido, Okechinyere Achilonu, Blessing Ogbuokiri, Chimeremma Sandra Amadi, Lawal Habeebullahi, Tony Ohalloran, Chidozine Williams Chukwu, Ebikella Domor Mienye, Mikail Aliyu, Olufunke Fasawe, Ibukunola Abosede Modupe, Erepamo Job Omietimi and Kehinde Aruleba, "An improved framework for detecting thyroid disease using filter-based feature selection and stacking ensemble," IEEE, 2024.

[18] L. Aversano, M. L. Bernardi, M. Cimitile, A. Maiellaro and R. Pecori, "A systematic review on artificial intelligence techniques for detecting thyroid diseases," *PeerJ Comput. Sci.*, vol.9, p. e1394, June, 2023.

[19] Stephanie S. Noronha, Mayuri A. Mehta, Dweepna Garg, Ketan Kotecha and Ajith Abraham, "Deep learning- based dermatological condition detection: a systematic review with recent methods, datasets, challenges, and future directions," IEEE, 2023.

[20] Y. Zhu, Y.-K. Wang, H.-P. Chen, K.-L. Gao, C. Shu, J.-C. Wang, L.-F. Yan, Y.-G. Yang, F.-Y. Xie, and J. Liu, "A deep learning based framework for diagnosing multiple skin diseases in a clinical environment," *Frontiers Med.*, vol. 8, April 2021, Art. no. 626369.

[21] Yu- Wei Chan, Tzu-Hsuan Huang, Yu-Tse Tsan, We-Chen Chan, Chih-Hung Chang, Yin-Te Tsai, "The risk classification of ergonomic musculoskeletal disorders in work-related repetitive manual handling operations with deep learning approaches," ICPAI, 2020.

[22] A. Klussmann, F. Liebers, H. Gebhardt, M. A. Rieger, U. Latza, and U. Steinberg, "Risk assessment of manual handling operations at work with the key indicator method (kim-mho)—determination of criterion validity regarding the prevalence of musculoskeletal symptoms and clinical conditions within a cross-sectional study," *BMC Musculoskeletal Disorders*, vol. 18, no. 1, p. 184, 2017.

Chapter 5

AI for Diseases Detection and Prevention

M T Vasumathi and Manju Sadasivan

5.1 Introduction

Nowadays, in most health fields, artificial intelligence (AI) technologies have been widely applied for the attainment of accurate insights into serious diseases and disorders. The ability of AI to process medical images efficiently has also been indispensable in diagnosing and making a prognosis in regard to diseases. Some of the key tools in effectively integrating AI into healthcare services include learning algorithms or large datasets derived from medical records or wearable devices. These tools enhance diagnoses and classifications of diseases, decision-making procedures, the performance of walking aids, and treatment, and finally ensure patient safety and longevity. AI accelerates medical analysis. For example, diagnosing tumors in images are early diagnoses that can be treated without taking long procedures in the lab. Finally, AI algorithms have uniquely talented skills in identifying undiagnosed and rare diseases, thereby providing excellent chances for early detection [1].

Machine learning (ML) and DL techniques are now being widely used for the diagnosis of heart disease. There are several imaging methods, such as CT, ECG, and echocardiography, that have DL facilities to analyze advanced cardiovascular data. Early diagnosis of coronary atherosclerotic heart disease, a common cardiovascular disorder, is crucial for its treatment. ML and DL have made remarkable strides in the diagnosis of this disease, where ML-based CT-Fractional Flow Reserve (CT-FFR) helps in a less complex, time-consuming process of diagnosis, thereby improving major adverse cardiac event predictions. In addition to this, AI applications have been serving in medical practices for the prediction and diagnosis of diseases of the

DOI: 10.1201/9781003617013-5

brain. Neurodegenerative diseases like Alzheimer's and Parkinson's are hard to identify, and recent ML and DL approaches have provided better diagnosis techniques.
Huge amounts of data related to the brain are processed by AI, which unfolds what
is not visible to a human. DL-based CNN models are preferred largely for disease
detection, which shows a great accuracy level in the prediction of diseases related to
Alzheimer's and Parkinson's. Another significant area that AI has contributed to is in
the early diagnosis and treatment of breast cancer, an attribute of death in women.
Algorithms such as LSSVM, fuzzy-artificial immune systems, and optimized SVMs
have been placed on very successful detection and prognosis of breast cancer cases
with accuracy levels that are excellent [2].

In the domain of genetic disorders, ML techniques like neural networks, random forests (RF), and support vector machines (SVMs) are useful for predictive and
classification purposes regarding genetic diseases. Though there are challenges in
developing biomarkers for complex genetic diseases, the use of AI techniques
enhances predictability. For instance, ANN-based models and supervised ML methods have also been applied successfully to classify cancerous microarray data as well
as to predict autism spectrum disorders.

AI techniques have been widely applied in the fields of dermatology in terms of
diagnosis, prediction, and classification of different skin-related disorders. The early
stages of skin cancer can be found through automated AI systems that do not rely
on human mistakes regarding patient outcomes. DL-based CNN algorithms are
largely used for the analysis of skin cancer lesions with high accuracy for prediction
and classification. Figure 5.1 shows the various application areas of AI/ML in
healthcare.

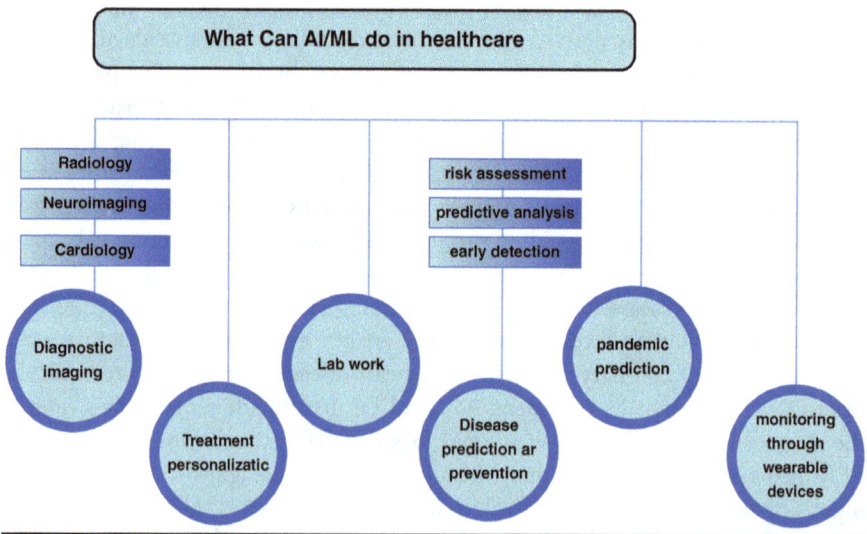

Figure 5.1   AI/ML in healthcare.

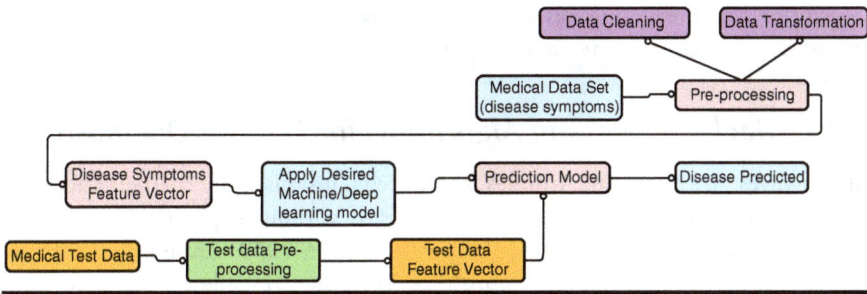

Figure 5.2   Detection process framework using ML.

In digital pathology, the addition of AI increases the correct rate of diagnosis concerning prostate cancer. AI-based technologies predict patient responses to both kinds of therapy. Furthermore, using the AI models, for instance, DL-based XmasNet, there has been a much greater accuracy reported in the classification of prostate cancer lesions.

Promising results have been achieved in the early detection of lung cancer through AI techniques, such as those based on CT and X-ray images. Early detection increases the survival rate, and based on this criterion, AI methods, such as DL-based frameworks, CNNs, and studies on comprehensive lung nodules, determine a high degree of accuracy in diagnosing and classifying lung cancer [3]. Figure 5.2 shows the general framework of the detection process using AI.

5.2 AI in Patient Diagnosis

Medical AI tries to design algorithms and methods to make an accurate disease diagnosis. Medical diagnosis concerns disease or syndrome definition through a clinical presentation of symptoms and signs, normally solicited from the patient's history and physical examination. It is indeed a very challenging process because the symptoms revolving around it are generally vague and can only be correctly diagnosed by practicing health professionals. In many countries, proper diagnostic procedures have faced great challenges in their delivery to the populations. Another drawback is that diagnostic tests are pricey and usually inaccessible to low-income people.

The increasing mistakes leading to misdiagnosis due to human error eventually result in overdiagnosis, thereby bringing together unwanted medical treatments and health and economic damages to patients. Some misdiagnoses might be caused by slight symptoms, rare diseases, or conditions being overlooked.

AI helps in making decisions and workflow management, as well as the automation of tasks. Advanced ML techniques have been used for purposes of triage, such as determining abnormalities in healthcare and setting priorities according to the severity of life-threatening cases. AI also helps physicians in diagnosing cardiac arrhythmia, stroke outcomes, and chronic diseases [4].

5.2.1 Machine Learning Algorithms for Disease Diagnosis

ML involves analyzing data samples to draw conclusions using mathematical and statistical methods, enabling machines to learn without explicit programming. Arthur Samuel first highlighted ML's significance in 1959 through his work on games and pattern recognition algorithms. The core principle of ML is to learn from data to make predictions or decisions based on the given task. ML technology allows many time-consuming tasks to be completed quickly and efficiently. With the exponential growth of computing power and data capacity, training data-driven ML models to predict outcomes with high accuracy has become increasingly feasible. Various papers outline different ML approaches, which are generally classified into three main categories: supervised, unsupervised, and semi-supervised learning. Additionally, ML algorithms can be subdivided based on different learning methods, including AdaBoost logistic regression, SVM, RF, and naïve Bayes (NB) [5].

5.2.1.1 AdaBoost Algorithm

AdaBoost (Adaptive Boosting) is an ensemble learning technique that enhances the performance of classifiers by creating a strong classifier from several weak classifiers. In disease detection using AdaBoost, the process begins with data acquisition, gathering medical data including patient diagnostics, symptoms, and history [6]. Data preprocessing follows, cleansing the data by handling outliers and missing values. Feature selection is then performed to identify relevant features impacting illness classification, often using algorithms like recursive feature elimination (RFE). The dataset is split into training and testing subsets, and initially, equal weights are assigned to all training instances. Multiple weak classifiers are trained iteratively, with misclassified instances' weights increasing after each iteration. These weak classifiers are then combined into a stronger model, with more weight given to better-performing classifiers. The final ensemble model's performance is assessed using metrics like accuracy and the confusion matrix. Finally, the trained AdaBoost model is deployed for real-time disease detection based on patient data. The AdaBoost algorithm technique is shown in Figure 5.3.

Applications of AdaBoost in disease detection include image classification, where it detects diseases through imaging data such as X-rays and magnetic resonance imaging (MRIs); risk prediction, classifying patients as high-risk or low-risk for specific diseases based on historical data; and cancer detection, enhancing the accuracy of cancer detection models by combining various features from biopsies and imaging.

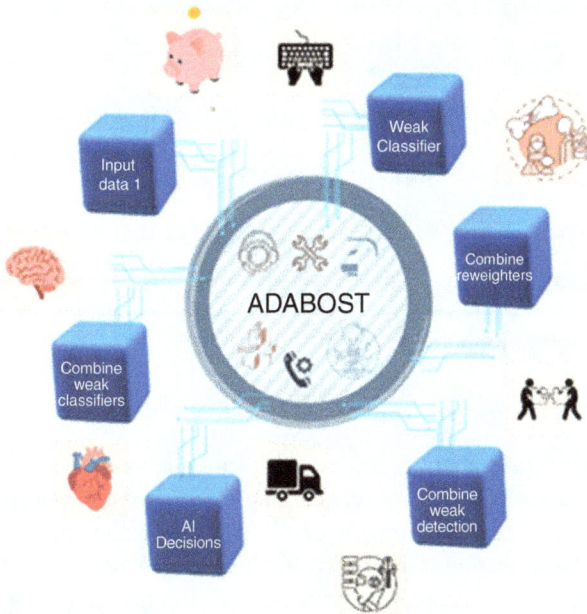

Figure 5.3   AdaBoost algorithm in disease detection.

5.2.1.2 Logistic Regression

Logistic regression is a statistical method used for binary classification in disease detection, predicting the probability of an event occurring, such as the presence or absence of a disease. The core component of logistic regression is the logit function, which transforms any real-valued number into a range between 0 and 1, representing the probability of the positive class. The sigmoid curve of logistic regression is shown in Figure 5.4. The cost function, or cross-entropy loss, is crucial for training the model and is defined as:

$$J(\theta) = -\frac{1}{m}\sum_{i=1}^{m}\left[y^{(i)}\log\left(h_\theta\left(x^{(i)}\right)\right) + \left(1 - y^{(i)}\right)\log\left(1 - h_\theta\left(x^{(i)}\right)\right)\right]$$

where $h_\theta(x)$ is the predicted probability calculated by the logistic function? $h_\theta(x) = \frac{1}{1 + e^{-\theta Tx}}$, $y^{(i)}$ is the actual label, and m is the number of training examples.

The cross-entropy loss measures how well the predicted probabilities match the actual outcomes by penalizing incorrect predictions. The goal is to minimize this cost function to optimize the model parameters, enhancing its ability to accurately classify and detect diseases based on input data [7].

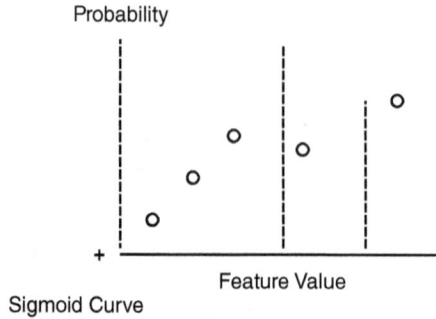

Figure 5.4   Logistic regression.

5.2.1.3 *Support Vector Machines*

The SVM algorithm is a strong supervised learning approach, widely used for the purpose of classification, which is very commonly employed for disease detection. It works on determining the optimal hyperplane in an N-dimensional space for differentiating between various classes of data. These data classes may somewhat resemble healthy and diseased samples. Steps associated with the method of application of SVM in disease detection The first step is data acquisition: This collects relevant information obtained from medical records, lab results, and imaging, such as age, blood pressure, and glucose levels. Following this is the data preprocessing stage, which cleans data concerning missing values and outliers by normalization or standardization of features to ensure uniformity throughout the dataset. Then feature selection is applied to find which attributes are the most useful ones for diagnosis, using algorithms such as RFE or Principal Component Analysis (PCA). The set is split into training and testing subsets, typically 70:30. In training, the SVM model gets tuned in order to determine the best hyperplane that maximizes the margin between classes. When necessary, kernels are used to map the data into higher dimensions: linear, polynomial, and RBF. The model is tested through performance metrics like accuracy, precision, recall, and F1-score on the testing set. Once cross-validated, the SVM model can be deployed in real-time; given new patient data, it determines the SVM class of the disease [8].

SVM is flexible and strong for the detection of disease, thereby making it very accurate and robust in the classification of complex data. SVM can continue to analyze the characteristics of the tumor from images or genomic data and will distinguish whether it is a benign or malignant tumor during a cancer diagnosis. In the case of diabetes prediction, SVM assesses several patient metrics in order to classify those prone to the disease. It further helps in the classification of heart disease by processing heart metrics, like ECG data, to predict probable heart conditions. SVM further helps in COVID-19 detection also, as it classifies chest X-rays or CT scans to see if there is a positive or negative infection with COVID-19. With operations like data preprocessing, model training, and evaluation, SVM helps healthcare professionals make the right decisions; therefore, health improvement, consistency, and better diagnostic analysis.

5.2.1.4 K-Nearest Neighbor (KNN)

One of these algorithms is K-Nearest Neighbor (KNN), which has been applied within non-parametric methods and classification and regression tasks. The application is of high utility in the detection of a disease because it classifies a sample by determining the majority class among the K-nearest neighbors in the feature space. First, the process begins with acquiring the data together with the relevant medical information, such as patient characteristics, lab results, and demographics. Data preprocessing includes the removal of duplicate entries, removal of missing values, and normalization for uniform contribution of features. Then feature selection is done to see which set of features is most pertinent to the disease. Data set is divided into training and testing in the ratio 70:30. The value of K, or the number of nearest neighbors, is chosen very carefully because a small K leads to noisy results while a large K may miss the local patterns; cross-validation often comes into use when finding the optimal K. Distances, as Euclidean, are calculated between instances in the testing set and those in the training set. The model gives a majority vote of K nearest training instances to label the class. It then checks the performance of this model in terms of accuracy and F1-score, and after validation, it deploys the KNN model in real time for the detection of disease based on incoming patient data [9].

Heart disease classification involves assessing patient metrics such as cholesterol levels and blood pressure to determine the risk of heart disease. Diabetes detection uses medical history and test results to classify individuals as diabetic or non-diabetic. Cancer detection focuses on identifying cancer types, such as benign or malignant, using tumor data and histopathological features.

5.2.1.5 Naive Bayes

The NB classifier is a probabilistic model grounded in Bayes' theorem, renowned for its effectiveness in text classification and also widely used in disease detection. The process begins with data acquisition, gathering relevant patient information such as medical records, symptoms, and lab results. Data preprocessing involves managing missing data and encoding categorical features, often through techniques like one-hot encoding. Feature selection is performed to identify the most predictive features using methods like chi-square tests. The dataset is then split into training and testing subsets. Probabilities are calculated for each class by determining prior probabilities (P(Class)) and likelihoods (P(Feature Class)). For new instances, Bayes' theorem is applied to compute posterior probabilities for each class, assigning the class with the highest probability. Figure 5.5 shows a model of NB used in disease detection. The model's performance is evaluated through classification accuracy and metrics such as

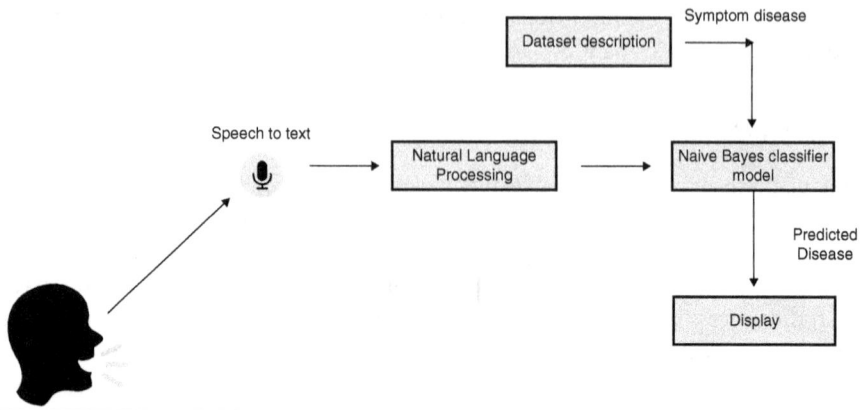

Figure 5.5   Naive Bayes for disease detection.

the confusion matrix. Finally, the trained NB model is deployed to predict disease presence in new patients based on their features [10].

Disease diagnosis involves classifying various diseases by analyzing symptoms and lab results to determine the presence of specific conditions. Risk assessment, on the other hand, evaluates the likelihood of patients developing certain conditions by examining their medical history and lifestyle factors.

5.3 Advanced AI Techniques for Disease Prevention

Computer vision and ML can significantly augment the traditional microscope work performed by pathologists. Machine vision is integral to diagnostic applications that assess physiological data, environmental factors, and genetic information. Clinicians now have access to extensive medical datasets, including symptoms, test results, and imaging files. Analyzing this rich resource enables a deeper understanding of biological mechanisms and risk factors [10].

AI enhances decision-making, workflow management, and task automation. In healthcare, ML is employed in triage to detect abnormalities and prioritize critical cases. AI also assists physicians in diagnosing cardiac arrhythmias, predicting stroke outcomes, and managing chronic diseases. Deep learning further contributes to various fields: in pathology, it helps diagnose diseases from lab results; in dermatology and oncology, it identifies cancerous tissue from biopsies; in genetic disorders, it aids in diagnosing rare diseases based on observed phenotypes; in facial analysis, it measures vital signs; and chatbots use text or speech recognition to detect patterns in patient symptoms, provide provisional diagnoses, and recommend treatments or actions.

5.3.1 Skin Cancer Detection and Prevention

AI, in the way it can improve early detection, treatment personalization, and monitoring of patients, is transforming skin cancer prevention. Deep learning models for AI algorithms can, for instance, analyze images of the skin to identify melanomas as well as other cancerous lesions with stunning precision that, in most cases, trumps human analysis. Predictive models based on AI assess a person's risk of contracting skin cancers using genetic markers of a person, skin type, and lifestyle. With AI, patient-specific, data-driven treatment plans are optimized to ensure that there is the best possible therapy outcome. The ML Model of skin cancer detection is shown in Figure 5.6. The use of AI-driven mobile apps allows for the remote monitoring of changes in the skin over time, thus enabling early identification of suspicious lesions. AI additionally helps in biopsy analysis by dermatologists and pathologists for more accurate diagnoses. Despite the challenges of being biased or integrated in a workflow-strict clinical environment, AI has revolutionized skin cancer prevention through early detection, individualized care, and long-term risk monitoring [11].

At Stanford University, researchers have developed a deep learning algorithm to diagnose skin cancer using convolutional neural networks (CNNs). Trained on a dataset of 130,000 images of skin lesions, covering over 2,000 different conditions, this ML model aims to enhance early detection, which is crucial for improving survival rates. Currently, US physicians diagnose about 5.4 million skin cancer cases annually through visual inspections with dermatoscopes and subsequent biopsies if needed. In tests, Stanford's algorithm demonstrated diagnostic precision comparable to that of 21 certified dermatologists examining 370 images. Although the results are promising, further validation is necessary before clinical deployment.

5.3.2 Cellular Pathology

For more than a century, traditional methodology in cellular pathology has been the mainstream diagnostic technique by visual inspection of the human pathologist on microscope images. Effective though it has still been cumbersome, labor-intensive,

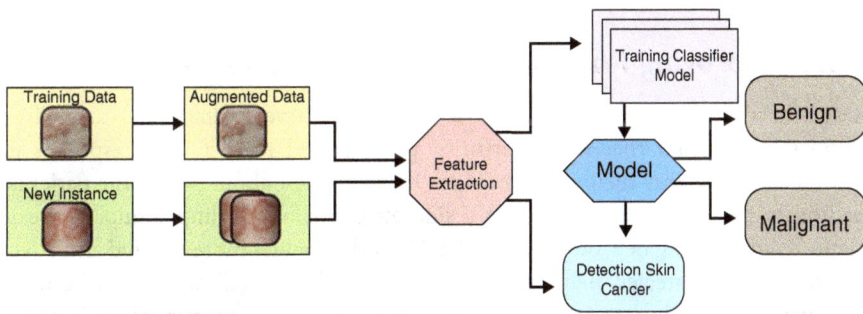

Figure 5.6   ML model for skin cancer detection.

and entirely judgmental on human pathologists' practice. Since the early years of the twentieth century, pathologists have played the critical role of classifying aberrant cell morphology or arrangement within tissue samples to make diagnoses, both basic such as infections and complex like cancers. However, this is also prone to human limitation factors, such as fatigue and variability in interpretation can on occasion affect the accuracy of diagnostics [12].

Recent advances in technological know-how, particularly in the fields of AI and ML, have presented them with a new horizon of modernizing pathology practices. In a seminal contribution in this direction, researchers at "Beth Israel Deaconess Medical Center" and "Harvard Medical School" leveraged deep learning—a form of ML modeled on the structure of the human brain—in assisting to classify and interpret hundreds of microscope scan results.

Being trained on these amounts of pathology data, the model was able to achieve a blindingly high diagnostic accuracy of 92%. Though this is slightly lower than the generally accepted 96% linked with an expert pathologist, it is still considered a major achievement for AI in medical diagnostics. One possible payoff of this algorithm's fast analysis of big volumes of scan data is to relieve the time lag put on pathologists so that preliminary assessment and prioritization of cases can be made faster.

More impressive, however, is the collaboration between human expertise and AI. When the deep learning model was factored with those of human pathologists' assessments, there was a gigantic leap in accuracy to a 99.5% rate. This significant advancement shows that though AI alone has not reached the level of human pathologists, it certainly is a very great assistant to supplement their work. In collaboration, AI and human pathologists can almost attain near-perfect diagnostic precision, thus giving fewer chances for the diagnosis to go wrong and better outcomes for the patients.

This human–machine partnership will therefore be the future of cellular pathology and diagnostic medicine. Deep learning combined with routine diagnosis promises enormous promise to deliver more accuracy, eradicate errors, and give patients faster, reliable diagnoses. As AI evolves, so will its roles in pathology and other medical fields, which are due to extend support to clinicians, ultimately improving healthcare delivery.

5.3.3 Improving Rheumatoid Arthritis Treatment

Researchers at Queen Mary University of London have leveraged AI to analyze blood samples from rheumatoid arthritis patients and predict their responses to treatment. Many anti-rheumatic drugs are ineffective for about half of the patients, leading to prolonged and unnecessary side effects before finding a suitable treatment. By identifying new biomarkers, the AI model enables more tailored and effective treatment strategies, helping doctors predict which medications will be most effective for individual patients and reducing the trial and error involved in treatment adjustments [13].

5.3.4 Using AI to Reduce the Risk of Heart Attacks

To minimize the risk of heart attacks, several applications connected to AI function towards increasing the chances of early detection, tailored care, and constant surveillance. Predictive models, built with the help of AI, can analyze patient health data like blood pressure, cholesterol, and genetics so that some high-risk individuals are identified in advance. Advanced analysis, including ECG and imaging, also allows for early diagnosis by detecting some subtle anomalies that might precede a heart attack. For instance, through wearable smartwatches, AI-driven platforms continuously monitor one's vital signs, alerting their users to potential problems in time. AI has also led to personalized treatment plans with optimized recommendations concerning medications and lifestyles according to an individual's needs. Next, through genomics and precision medicine, prevention is enhanced further as the specific genetic markers associated with heart disease are identified. The patients' data, which was gathered from different sources, are fed to AI systems for immediate in vivo alerts on slight signs of medical deterioration, thereby making it impleadable in hospital settings. While data privacy and clinical validation are some of the issues in implementing AI systems in healthcare, it is full of promise regarding heart attack prevention through better prediction, monitoring, and treatment [14].

Here's a diagram illustrating these AI applications for reducing heart attack risks (Figure 5.7).

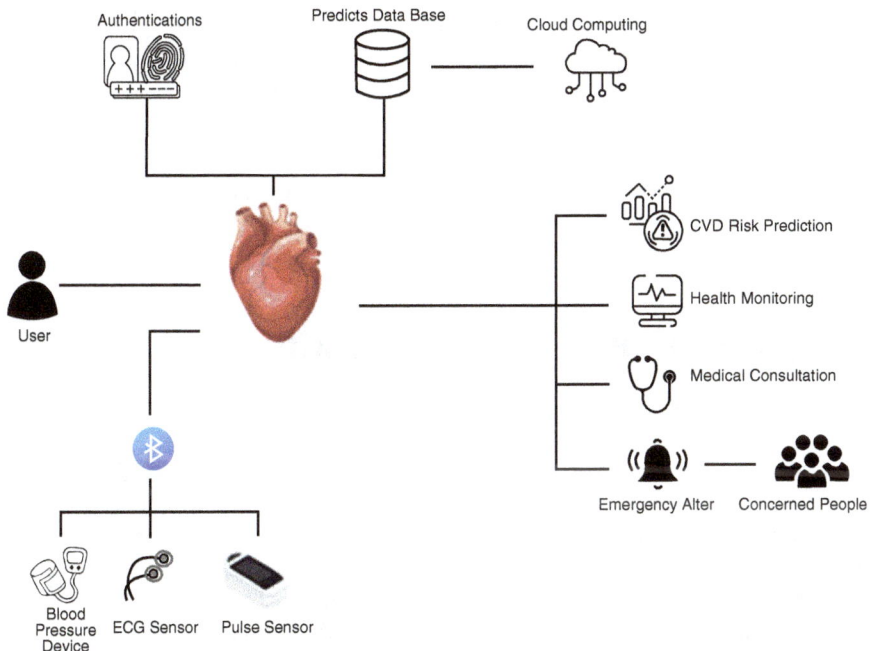

Figure 5.7 AI framework for heart attack prevention.

5.4 AI in Medical Imaging: X-Rays, MRIs, and CT Scans

Advancements in medical imaging and AI have ushered in a transformative era in healthcare, reshaping early disease detection, diagnosis, treatment planning, and patient outcomes. Medical imaging techniques such as computed tomography (CT), MRI, and positron emission tomography (PET) provide detailed visual data of the human body, generating vast amounts of information that AI efficiently analyzes.

AI, particularly through deep learning algorithms, excels at uncovering valuable insights from medical images. These models, trained on extensive datasets, can identify intricate patterns and features that might not be visible to the human eye, enhancing diagnostic precision and efficiency. AI supports healthcare professionals by detecting abnormalities, identifying specific structures, and predicting disease outcomes.

By leveraging ML, AI systems analyze medical images with remarkable speed and accuracy, facilitating early disease detection that traditional methods might miss. This early identification is crucial for timely treatment, potentially saving lives and improving patient outcomes [14].

AI also advances image segmentation and quantification, enabling accurate identification of structures like tumors, blood vessels, or cells. This capability is vital for precise treatment planning, optimizing surgical procedures, and delivering targeted therapies.

Furthermore, AI contributes to personalized medicine by analyzing medical images and patient data to create individualized treatment plans. This tailored approach enhances treatment effectiveness and minimizes side effects, improving overall patient care.

In surgical settings, AI enhances image-guided interventions by combining pre-operative imaging with real-time data. This integration provides surgeons with improved visualization, navigation support, and decision-making tools, leading to greater precision, reduced risks, and more minimally invasive procedures.

5.5 Enhancing Patient Outcomes with AI

The US Institute of Medicine has highlighted that diagnostic errors contribute to about 10% of patient deaths and a similar proportion of treatment complications. These errors are not necessarily due to the performance of medical professionals but often arise from systemic issues such as communication breakdowns, fragmented healthcare IT systems, and computers that fail to support proper procedures. Addressing these issues, AI plays a crucial role in enhancing the efficiency and accuracy of medical practice. By supporting clinical staff, AI helps alleviate burnout caused by excessive workloads and exhaustion, providing valuable assistance in managing tasks and streamlining workflows.

Recent advancements in healthcare computer systems have significantly improved the efficiency of image management. For example, radiologists can now handle and analyze numerous images with greater ease, leading to improved diagnostic capacity and accuracy. This efficiency allows specialists to quickly review and flag critical scanner images, enabling them to address urgent cases more effectively and promptly.

Beyond diagnostic improvements, ML has transformative impacts on various aspects of healthcare. In drug development and trials, ML accelerates the discovery of new drugs and optimizes trial designs. In clinical research, it enhances data analysis and helps identify promising treatment pathways. In robotic surgery, ML contributes to innovations such as automatic suturing, which can shorten surgery durations and reduce surgeon fatigue, thereby improving overall surgical outcomes [15].

5.5.1 Predictive Analytics for Patient Health Outcomes

Predictive analytics is essential in healthcare for improving care delivery and patient outcomes. By analyzing historical data, health systems can anticipate future events from both operational and clinical perspectives. This capability is particularly beneficial for healthcare organizations committed to value-based care, as forecasting outcomes enables stakeholders to pinpoint deficiencies in their current strategies and make necessary adjustments. This method is especially relevant to risk stratification and chronic disease management, where effective implementation can greatly reduce adverse outcomes and associated costs (Figure 5.8).

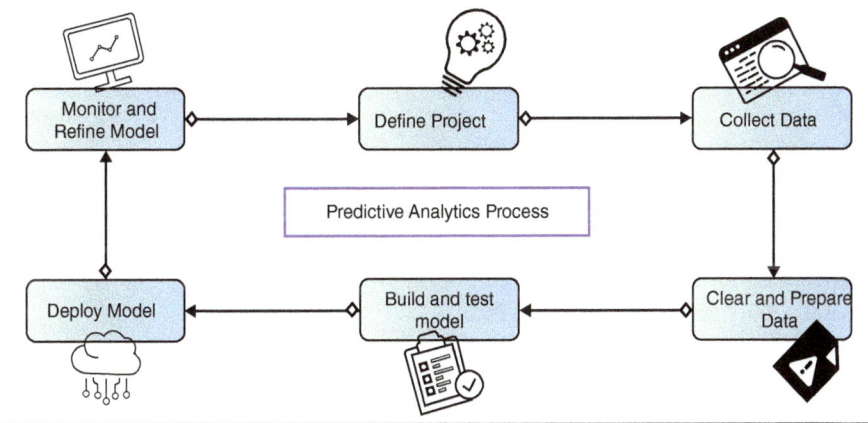

Figure 5.8 Predictive analytics process flow for patient health outcomes.

5.5.1.1 Enhancing Clinical Decision Making

One of the most significant applications of healthcare predictive analytics is in supporting clinical decisions. Effective risk scoring enhances clinical decision-making by pinpointing risk factors within a patient population, enabling health systems to mitigate risks effectively. These scores are created by identifying relevant risk factors for adverse events, such as a family history of high blood pressure, and analyzing their impact on a patient's risk. The scores are then integrated into risk-scoring models that aggregate data from multiple sources to stratify risk on both individual and population levels.

Risk scoring and stratification have numerous applications in healthcare, including aiding care teams in forecasting disease progression or treatment success. This is particularly valuable in chronic disease management, where structured treatment plans help patients manage their conditions and improve their quality of life. Predictive analytics can quickly evaluate treatment efficacy, guiding clinicians on whether to adjust a patient's care plan or continue with the current therapy.

Patients' responses to different treatments can vary, posing a challenge for clinicians. To address this, researchers at the University of Michigan Rogel Cancer Center developed a predictive model for patients with HPV-positive throat cancer. This model forecasts treatment effectiveness months earlier than standard imaging scans, overcoming the issue of pseudo-progression, where successful treatment initially causes a tumor to grow before shrinking. The model provides a blood test to determine treatment efficacy after a single cycle.

Predictive analytics allows healthcare professionals to analyze data swiftly and plan the most effective treatments, saving time and improving outcomes [16].

5.5.1.2 Advancing Population Health Management

Beyond clinical decision support, predictive analytics is vital for population health management. Predictive modeling enables healthcare stakeholders to monitor care trends, such as disease prevalence and comorbidities, within a patient population. This data supports efforts to manage population health, such as preventing hospital readmissions and promoting preventive care.

Predictive analytics is increasingly important for coordinating care for populations disproportionately affected by climate change. The climate crisis poses significant public health threats, including increased costs related to illnesses, injuries, and premature death, which strain health systems, especially during climate-related disasters like hurricanes and wildfires.

5.5.1.3 Improving Value-Based Care Implementation

Clinical decision support and population health management are crucial for a healthcare organization's value-based care strategy. Effective use of predictive analytics can enhance patient and provider engagement, alleviating some challenges in transitioning to value-based care.

Payers and providers use predictive modeling to enhance care coordination efforts. Predictive modeling identifies high-risk members, enabling targeted outreach and care coordination.

Predictive analytics help stakeholders assess risks like unplanned admissions, heart failure, and pneumonia, creating risk-based patient cohorts for better care management.

5.6 Genomics and AI

AI and ML are increasingly pivotal in genomics, revolutionizing how we analyze and interpret complex genetic data. Below are detailed applications of AI/ML in genomics:

Facial Analysis for Genetic Disorders: AI-powered facial recognition tools are being used to diagnose genetic disorders by analyzing facial features. These systems are trained on extensive datasets containing images of individuals with known genetic conditions. The AI algorithms detect subtle facial dysmorphisms that are characteristic of certain genetic syndromes. For example:

Algorithm Training: AI models are trained using thousands of facial images from patients with genetic disorders, creating a database of facial features associated with specific conditions.

Diagnostic Application: When a new patient's image is input into the system, the AI compares their facial features with the database, identifying potential genetic disorders. For instance, a facial recognition algorithm might identify features indicative of conditions like Noonan syndrome or Williams syndrome.

Early Detection: By identifying these features early, the AI aids in prompt diagnosis and intervention, potentially improving patient outcomes and enabling early treatment strategies.

Cancer Type Identification from Liquid Biopsies: Liquid biopsies, which analyze biomarkers in blood samples, are increasingly used for cancer detection and monitoring. AI and ML enhance this process by:

Data Integration: ML models analyze a combination of genetic, epigenetic, and proteomic data obtained from liquid biopsies. This includes evaluating levels of circulating tumor DNA (ctDNA), RNA, or proteins.

Classification Algorithms: AI algorithms classify the type of cancer based on patterns in the biomarker data. For example, ML models can differentiate between breast cancer subtypes or identify the presence of lung cancer by comparing biomarker profiles against known cancer signatures.

Clinical Impact: This approach provides a non-invasive method for identifying cancer types, which is crucial for early diagnosis, monitoring treatment response, and adjusting therapeutic strategies [17].

Cancer Progression Prediction: AI/ML models predict cancer progression by analyzing various data sources:

Historical Data Analysis: ML algorithms analyze historical patient data, including genomic information, tumor characteristics, treatment history, and patient demographics.

Predictive Modeling: Algorithms use this data to build predictive models that forecast the likelihood of cancer progression, metastasis, or recurrence. For instance, survival analysis models might predict the time to relapse or the probability of metastatic spread.

Clinical Use: These predictions help oncologists personalize treatment plans, choose appropriate therapies, and make informed decisions about patient management, potentially improving outcomes and reducing unnecessary treatments.

Identifying Disease-Causing Genomic Variants: AI tools help distinguish between pathogenic and benign genetic variants:

Variant Classification: ML algorithms are trained to recognize patterns associated with pathogenic variants by analyzing large-scale genomic datasets and clinical records.

Integration with Databases: AI models integrate information from various genetic databases and literature to assess the clinical significance of variants. For example, a variant identified in a patient's genome can be cross-referenced with known disease-associated variants to determine its pathogenicity.

Clinical Implications: Accurate classification of variants is crucial for genetic counseling and personalized medicine, helping to identify individuals at risk of genetic disorders and guiding treatment options.

Enhancing Gene Editing: Tools Deep learning improves gene editing technologies like CRISPR by:

Predictive Modeling: AI models predict the effectiveness and specificity of CRISPR guide RNAs by analyzing genomic sequences and previous editing outcomes. These predictions help design more accurate and efficient CRISPR systems.

Off-Target Prediction: Deep learning algorithms assess potential off-target effects by modeling the interactions between CRISPR components and the genome, reducing the risk of unintended genetic modifications.

Optimization: AI tools assist in optimizing guide RNA sequences and delivery methods, making gene editing more precise and reducing potential side effects.

Predicting Viral Genomic Variations: AI/ML models anticipate future variations in viral genomes, such as those of influenza and SARS-CoV-2:

Mutation Tracking: ML algorithms analyze historical genomic data from viral strains to identify mutation patterns and predict future variations.

Modeling Evolution: AI models simulate viral evolution based on observed mutation rates and environmental factors, providing insights into potential future strains.

Public Health Applications: This predictive capability aids in vaccine development and epidemic preparedness by anticipating changes in viral genomes and informing public health strategies.

AI and ML are transforming genomics by providing sophisticated tools for analyzing and interpreting genetic data. These technologies enhance diagnostic accuracy, optimize treatment strategies, and contribute to public health efforts. As AI/ML technologies continue to advance, they hold promise for even greater breakthroughs in understanding genetic diseases and developing personalized medicine [18].

5.6.1 Natural Language Processing in Healthcare

One of the noteworthy AI technologies making progress in disease detection is natural language processing (NLP). It is possible to make use of NLP algorithms to retrieve significant clinical information from electronic health records (EHRs), medical literature, and patient reports. Unstructured data can be analyzed using NLP algorithms. This feature enables the identification of disease patterns and the prediction of potential outbreaks. Thus, NLP enhances the ability of healthcare providers to diagnose and manage diseases effectively.

A healthcare chatbot is an AI-powered software tool created to mimic conversations with human users, particularly in the healthcare setting, to offer information, assistance, or access to services. These chatbots employ NLP and ML to comprehend and respond to user inquiries, providing information that includes symptom checking and healthcare tips. Chatbots are ideally suited for telemedicine, providing a seamless interface for remote healthcare services. They can support remote patient monitoring, symptom tracking, and follow-up care, thereby increasing the reach and effectiveness of telemedicine [19]. Integrating chatbots into telemedicine signifies a major advancement in delivering accessible and efficient remote healthcare. Implementing healthcare chatbots requires addressing various ethical considerations and adhering to best practices for effective and responsible use. Healthcare providers must comply with privacy regulations such as HIPAA and GDPR, particularly regarding data collection and storage. Chatbots should be designed with strong security measures to protect patient data from breaches and unauthorized access.

5.7 Wearable Technology and AI

AI-powered wearable devices are transforming industries and everyday life. AI enhances the functionality and user experience of wearables by enabling features such as health monitoring, activity tracking, and personalized recommendations. By analyzing sensor data, AI algorithms offer insights and alerts that improve fitness tracking, health monitoring, and the overall convenience of wearable devices. Figure 5.9 depicts key examples of wearable AI devices.

Flexible electronics-based wearable health technology has recently garnered significant attention for patient health monitoring. This advancement offers the potential for early disease detection and prompt treatment. Wearable sensors have introduced a new dimension to personalized health monitoring by precisely tracking physical conditions and biochemical signals. Despite the advancements in wearable sensor technology, challenges remain in data accuracy, precise disease diagnosis, and early treatment. To address these issues, further progress is needed in applied materials and structures, along with the integration of AI-enabled wearable sensors. These improvements will help extract specific signals for precise clinical decision-making and more effective medical care [20]. Figure 5.10 illustrates how AI in wearable medical devices and fitness trackers has revolutionized the healthcare industry.

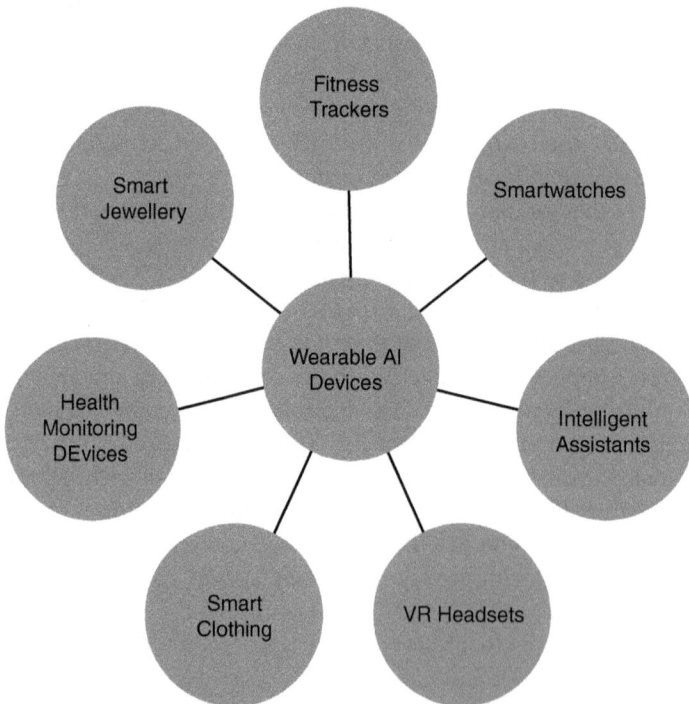

Figure 5.9   Wearable AI devices.

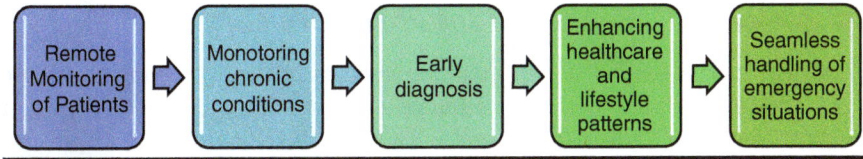

Figure 5.10 Ways in which AI wearable devices revolutionized the healthcare industry.

5.7.1 Health Monitoring through Wearable Devices

Wearable sensors can monitor a wide range of health parameters, including heart rate, blood pressure, oxygen saturation, skin temperature, physical activity, sleep patterns, and biochemical markers like glucose, cortisol, lactates, electrolytes, and pH, as well as environmental factors. This technology encompasses both first-generation devices, such as fitness trackers and smartwatches, as well as modern wearable sensors, making it a powerful tool for tackling healthcare challenges. The integration of IoT, cloud computing, and AI has aided researchers in diagnosing diabetes and heart disease. In this context, wearable sensors functioned as IoT devices to collect data, while AI techniques were utilized to process this data for disease diagnosis [21].

5.7.2 AI in Detecting Early Symptoms of Diseases

The data gathered by wearable sensors can be analyzed with ML and AI algorithms to offer insights into an individual's health, facilitating early detection of health issues and personalized healthcare. A major benefit of AI-based wearable health technology is its promotion of preventive healthcare, allowing individuals and healthcare providers to address symptomatic conditions proactively before they worsen. Additionally, wearable devices can motivate healthy behaviors by providing reminders and feedback on activities such as staying active, hydrating, eating health-ily, and maintaining a healthy lifestyle by measuring hydration biomarkers and nutrients.

AI algorithms can analyze the vast amounts of data collected by wearable devices, allowing healthcare providers to identify patterns, predict health outcomes, and make informed decisions about patient care. AI algorithms can analyze an individual's activity level, sleep patterns, and heart rate to predict the likelihood of heart attacks or strokes, enabling healthcare providers to take proactive measures. An AI-based disease detection system can predict the onset of diseases using patient records, genetic data, and lifestyle factors. Additionally, these algorithms can foresee complications from diseases like diabetes, such as detecting retinopathy from retinal images [22].

5.7.3 Health Data Analysis for Preventive Care

Preventive care is essential for maintaining good health and lowering healthcare costs. Historically, it has been reactive and generalized, without personalization and precision. However, with advancements in data analysis and technology, we are now on the verge of a healthcare revolution.

Predictive analytics, a powerful branch of data analysis, assists healthcare professionals in identifying potential health issues early on. By leveraging historical patient data and advanced algorithms, predictive analytics can detect subtle signs and symptoms that may signal an elevated risk of developing a specific condition. Early detection enables timely interventions, leading to better treatment outcomes and lower healthcare costs. Data analysis helps identify potential health risks and conditions at an early stage when they are more easily treatable. By examining individual patient data, healthcare providers can customize preventive care strategies to address specific risk factors, genetic predispositions, and lifestyle habits. Data analysis enables healthcare providers to efficiently allocate resources by identifying high-risk individuals needing immediate attention, thereby optimizing preventive care efforts. Proactive preventive care minimizes the need for complex and costly treatments by addressing health issues before they worsen, leading to substantial cost savings for both patients and healthcare systems (Figure 5.11).

The potential of data analysis in preventive care is vast. As technology advances, we can anticipate significant progress in this field, providing unprecedented opportunities to improve preventive care practices. AI can analyze complex healthcare data and detect patterns that might be overlooked by humans alone. Integrating AI algorithms into data analysis will enhance the accuracy and efficiency of preventive care. Additionally, advancements in genomics, when combined with data analysis, will enable more precise identification of individuals at risk for certain diseases, leading to tailored preventive care strategies. With the growing use of wearable devices and IoT-connected sensors, continuous remote monitoring will become more accessible and widespread, facilitating proactive preventive interventions [23].

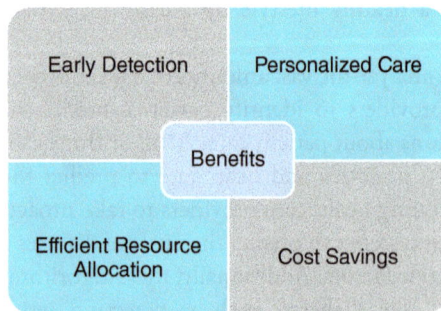

Figure 5.11   Benefits of data analysis in preventive care.

5.8 Case Studies and Real-World Applications

5.8.1 AI in Radiology—Detecting Breast Cancer

The integration of AI into radiology has revolutionized the detection and diagnosis of breast cancer. This case study examines the application of AI in mammogram interpretation, focusing on how it enhances efficiency and accuracy, ultimately improving patient outcomes.

Case Description: Traditionally, highly skilled radiologists are responsible for interpreting breast images. They are experts in selecting appropriate imaging techniques and thoroughly assessing patients' anatomy and any detected abnormalities or pathologies. When a woman undergoes a mammogram or other breast imaging, the radiologist meticulously describes each finding, including its location, size, shape, and density. However, human interpretation, while highly skilled, can be subjective and time-consuming, sometimes leading to variability in diagnoses [24].

Solution or Intervention: AI algorithms, particularly CNN, have the potential to significantly streamline and enhance the radiologist's workflow. These algorithms provide quantitative analyses that are not subject to human bias, enabling more consistent and objective interpretations of mammograms. AI-powered software can automate the interpretation of breast mammograms, ultrasounds, and MRI scans, allowing patients to receive their results more quickly [25].

Dataset: For this case study, we utilized the Digital Database for Screening Mammography (DDSM), which includes over 2,600 cases comprising normal, benign, and malignant findings. The dataset provides mammogram images with corresponding annotations for each case, serving as an excellent resource for training and evaluating AI models.

Methodology: The AI model used for this study is a CNN-based architecture, specifically ResNet-50, pre-trained on the ImageNet dataset and fine-tuned using the DDSM dataset. The training process involved splitting the dataset into training (70%), validation (15%), and testing (15%) sets. The model was trained to identify and classify abnormalities such as masses and calcifications.

The results obtained from the above methodology indicate that the AI model achieved high accuracy, sensitivity, and specificity in detecting breast cancer from mammogram images. The model's sensitivity (92%) reflects its ability to correctly identify positive cases, while its specificity (95%) indicates its effectiveness in correctly identifying negative cases. The precision (93%) and F1 score (92.5%) further demonstrate the model's balanced performance.

Comparative Analysis: When compared to human radiologists, the AI model demonstrated several advantages:

i) *Consistency*: The AI model provided consistent results across different cases, reducing the variability often seen in human interpretations.

    ii) *Speed*: The automated analysis significantly reduced the time required to interpret mammograms, allowing for quicker diagnosis and treatment.

    iii) *Detection of Subtle Abnormalities*: The AI model was able to detect subtle abnormalities and ambiguous features that might be missed by human eyes, leading to earlier detection of breast cancer [26].

Case Study Example: One case involved a 45-year-old woman with dense breast tissue. The AI model identified a small, subtle mass that was initially missed by the radiologist. Further analysis confirmed the mass as malignant, and early intervention was initiated. This case highlights the AI model's capability to enhance detection in challenging scenarios.

The application of AI in breast cancer detection showcases its transformative potential in enhancing screening accuracy and efficiency. The CNN-based model demonstrated high performance in detecting breast cancer from mammogram images, providing unbiased and objective analyses. By integrating AI into the diagnostic process, healthcare providers can deliver more precise, efficient, and tailored breast cancer care, ultimately saving lives and improving outcomes. Future research should focus on validating these tools across diverse populations, ensuring data standardization, and addressing regulatory and ethical considerations.

5.9 Conclusion

AI and ML enhance various aspects of health assessment, including disease prediction, diagnosis, and effective treatment. AI-enabled wearable health technology has immense potential to transform healthcare, revolutionizing how we monitor and manage our well-being. These advanced devices continuously track diverse health parameters, providing users with personalized insights and feedback. As technology progresses, AI-enabled wearable health devices can drive a shift in healthcare towards a more preventive and proactive approach. By offering personalized, continuous monitoring and remote patient care, these devices empower individuals to make proactive health choices, prevent potential complications, and alleviate the burden on healthcare systems.

References

1. Wani SUD, Khan NA, Thakur G, Gautam SP, Ali M, Alam P, Alshehri S, Ghoneim MM, Shakeel F. Utilization of Artificial Intelligence in Disease Prevention: Diagnosis, Treatment, and Implications for the Healthcare Workforce. *Healthcare* 2022;10(4):608. https://doi.org/10.3390/healthcare10040608
2. Thakur GK, Khan N, Anush H, Thakur A. AI-Driven Predictive Models for Early Disease Detection and Prevention. *2024 International Conference on Knowledge Engineering and Communication Systems (ICKECS)*, Chikkaballapur, India, 2024, pp. 1–6, doi: 10.1109/ICKECS61492.2024.10616851

3. Pierre K, Haneberg AG, Kwak S, Peters KR, Hochhegger B, Sananmuang T, Tunlayadechanont P, Tighe PJ, Mancuso A, Forghani R. Applications of Artificial Intelligence in the Radiology Roundtrip: Process Streamlining. *Workflow Optimization, and Beyond, Seminars in Roentgenology* 2023;58(2):158–169, ISSN 0037-198X, https://doi.org/10.1053/j.ro.2023.02.003

4. Al-Antari MA. Artificial Intelligence for Medical Diagnostics-Existing and Future AI Technology! *Diagnostics (Basel)* 2023 Feb 12;13(4):688. doi: 10.3390/diagnostics13040688. PMID: 36832175; PMCID: PMC9955430.

5. Ibrahim I, Abdulazeez A. Ibrahim Mahmood Ibrahim Adnan Mohsin Abdulazeez The Role of Machine Learning Algorithms for Diagnosing Diseases. *Journal of Applied Science and Technology Trends* 2021;2(01):10–19. https://doi.org/10.38094/jastt20179

6. Ganachari S, Battula SR. Stroke Disease Prediction Using Adaboost Ensemble Learning Technique. In H Sharma, V Shrivastava, KK Bharti, L Wang (Eds.), *Communication and Intelligent Systems. ICCIS 2022.* Lecture Notes in Networks and Systems (Vol. 686). Springer, 2023. https://doi.org/10.1007/978-981-99-2100-3_21

7. Asadi F, Rahmani AM, Darwesh RM. Heart Disease Detection Using Machine Learning Algorithms: A Logistic Regression Approach. *Journal of Biomedical Engineering and Informatics* 2023;12(3):145–158.

8. Hameed B, Al-Azawi A, Ali M. Anomaly Detection in Human Disease: A Hybrid Approach Using GWO-SVM for Gene Selection. *International Journal of Environmental Technology and Applied Science* 2023;34(2):14–22.

9. Muhammad Y, Tahir M, Hayat M, Chong KT. Heart Disease Prediction Using a Weighted K-Nearest Neighbor Algorithm. *Operations Research Forum* 2023;4(2):15–25.

10. Miranda E, Charankumar G, Dasore A. Detection of Cardiovascular Disease Risk Level for Adults Using Naive Bayes Classifier. *Healthcare Informatics Research* 2023;23(3):196–202. https://doi.org/10.4258/hir.2016.22.3.196

11. Luo N, Zhong X, Luxin S, Cheng Z, Ma W, Hao P. Artificial Intelligence-Assisted Dermatology Diagnosis: From Unimodal to Multimodal. *Computers in Biology and Medicine* 2023; 165:107413. ISSN 0010-4825, https://doi.org/10.1016/j.compbiomed.2023.107413

12. Hanna MG, Hanna MH. Current Applications and Challenges of Artificial Intelligence in Pathology. *Human Pathology Reports.*

13. Abbas S, Ojo S, Al Hejaili A et al. Artificial Intelligence Framework for Heart Disease Classification from Audio Signals. *Sci Rep* 2024;14:3123. https://doi.org/10.1038/s41598-024-53778-7

14. Pinto-Coelho L. How Artificial Intelligence Is Shaping Medical Imaging Technology: A Survey of Innovations and Applications. *Bioengineering (Basel)* 2023 Dec 18;10(12):1435. doi: 10.3390/bioengineering10121435. PMID: 38136026; PMCID: PMC10740686.

15. Kumar K, Kumar P, Deb D, Unguresan ML, Muresan V. Artificial Intelligence and Machine Learning Based Intervention in Medical Infrastructure: A Review and Future Trends. *Healthcare (Basel)* 2023 Jan 10;11(2):207. doi: 10.3390/healthcare11020207. PMID: 36673575; PMCID: PMC9859198.

16. https://www.foreseemed.com/predictive-analytics-in-healthcare

17. Connal S, Cameron JM, Sala A, Brennan PM, Palmer DS, Palmer JD, Perlow H, Baker MJ. Liquid Biopsies: The Future of Cancer Early Detection. *J Transl Med.* 2023 Feb 11;21(1):118. doi: 10.1186/s12967-023-03960-8. PMID: 36774504; PMCID: PMC9922467.

18. Abdallah S, Sharifa M, Almadhoun MK, Khawar Sr MM, Shaikh U, Balabel KM, Saleh I, Manzoor A, Mandal AK, Ekomwereren O, Khine WM. The Impact of Artificial Intelligence on Optimizing Diagnosis and Treatment Plans for Rare Genetic Disorders. *Cureus* 2023 Oct 11;15(10):e46860. doi: 10.7759/cureus.46860. PMID: 37954711; PMCID: PMC10636514.

19. Xu L, Sanders L, Li K, Chow JCL. Chatbot for Health Care and Oncology Applications Using Artificial Intelligence and Machine Learning: Systematic Review. *JMIR Cancer* 2021 Nov 29;7(4):e27850. doi: 10.2196/27850. PMID: 34847056; PMCID: PMC8669585.

20. Shajari S, Kuruvinashetti K, Komeili A, Sundararaj U. The Emergence of AI-Based Wearable Sensors for Digital Health Technology: A Review. *Sensors (Basel)* 2023 Nov 29;23(23):9498. doi: 10.3390/s23239498. PMID: 38067871; PMCID: PMC10708748.

21. Shajari S, Kuruvinashetti K, Komeili A, Sundararaj U. The Emergence of AI-Based Wearable Sensors for Digital Health Technology: A Review. *Sensors* 2023;23(23):9498. https://doi.org/10.3390/s23239498

22. Javaid M, Haleem A, Singh RP, Suman R, Rab S. Significance of Machine Learning in Healthcare: Features, Pillars and Applications. *International Journal of Intelligent Networks* 2022;3:58–73, ISSN 2666-6030, https://doi.org/10.1016/j.ijin.2022.05.002

23. https://moldstud.com/articles/p-the-impact-of-healthcare-data-analysis-on-preventive-care

24. Al-Karawi D, Al-Zaidi S, Helael KA, Obeidat N, Mouhsen AM, Ajam T, Alshalabi BA, Salman M, Ahmed MH. A Review of Artificial Intelligence in Breast Imaging. *Tomography* 2024;10(5):705–726. https://doi.org/10.3390/tomography10050055

25. Chauhan, A.S., Singh, R., Priyadarshi, N. et al. Unleashing the power of advanced technologies for revolutionary medical imaging: pioneering the healthcare frontier with artificial intelligence. Discov Artif Intell 4, 58 (2024). https://doi.org/10.1007/s44163-024-00161-0

26. Ahn JS, Shin S, Yang SA, Park EK, Kim KH, Cho SI, Ock CY, Kim S. Artificial Intelligence in Breast Cancer Diagnosis and Personalized Medicine. J Breast Cancer. 2023 Oct;26(5):405–435. doi: 10.4048/jbc.2023.26.e45. PMID: 37926067; PMCID: PMC10625863

Chapter 6

Machine Learning Techniques for Detecting Lung Cancer

Abhilasha Chauhan, Suchi Johari and Nishant Mathur

6.1 Introduction

6.1.1 Overview of Lung Cancer Detection and Its Significance

Lung cancer is a deadly cancer and can occur in the trachea, large airways, or lungs. This results from certain lungs' unchecked expansion and diffusion. Lung cancer is more likely to strike those who have a history of lung illness or chest conditions like emphysema. Excessive use of tobacco products, including cigarettes, is a significant risk factor for breast cancer among Indian men. However, the lower rate of smoking among Indian women suggests that there are other factors that contribute to the cancer in this group. Occupational chemicals, contaminants in the air, and gas radon inhalation are further dangers. Primary lung cancer and secondary lung cancer are two different types of cancer that emerge in the lungs or spread there from other parts of the body [1]. The overall dimension of the tumor and the severity of its transmission determine the cancer's stage. Early-stage cancers are small and confined to the lungs, while late-stage cancers have spread to other tissues or other parts of the body. An improved knowledge of the dangers can aid in the prevention of cancer. Early detection is critical to improving survival rates, and using machine learning (ML) technology to make the diagnostic process more efficient is critical to improving early detection [2, 3].

DOI: 10.1201/9781003617013-6   **117**

Lung cancer data utilized in this study came from Data World and the UCI ML Repository. Using the k-fold cross-validation approach, the data were divided into training and testing categories. Based on the data, classification models are constructed using methods such as logistic regression (LR), naïve Bayes (NB), support vector machines (SVM), and decision trees. These models are evaluated using test data to determine their accuracy [4, 5]. In the final step, the accuracy of each classification model is compared to determine its performance (Figure 6.1).

One million people lose their lives to lung cancer each decade, making it one of the most fatal diseases. As the incidence of pulmonary nodules increases, identifying nodules on chest CT has become important in modern medicine. Thus, it is critical to implement software-assisted detection, that is, CAD technologies, to guarantee early lung cancer diagnosis. The use of X-rays is used to obtain pictures of the human anatomy from all directions during a CT scan. Computers then analyze these photos to produce fine-grained pictures of the inside organs and tissues of the body.

6.1.2 Importance of Early Detection

According to the American Cancer Society, there were over 224,000 new cases in 2016 of cancer and 158,000 deaths from cancer, which is a significant problem, especially since the current 5-year survival rate is only 18%. This number is low

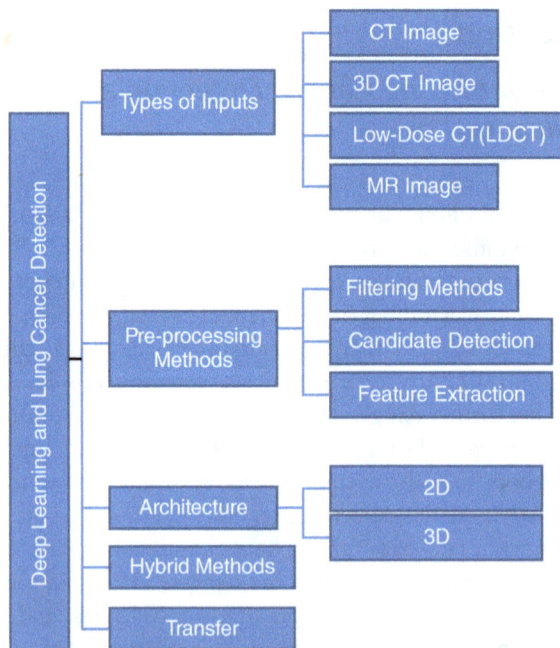

Figure 6.1   Overview of Deep Learning Techniques for Lung Cancer Detection.

compared to other cancers such as breast, colon, and prostate cancer, where modern screening has helped to increase the 5-year survival rate to 91%, 66%, and 99%, respectively. It is now clear that early detection of lung cancer saves lives. Unfortunately, most lung cancer diagnoses occur after symptoms begin, when the disease is usually at a higher stage and limits the opportunities for treatment. Effective early screening has long been needed to reduce the incidence of lung cancer [6, 7]. Procedures such as sputum cytology, chest X-ray, and CT scanning have been reviewed. The current recommendations for yearly LDCT screening for populations at increased risk stem from the National Lung Screening Trial (NLST), which demonstrated that LDCT screening reduced the rate of lung cancer by 20%. Efforts are underway to expand this screening process from the research setting to general clinical use to achieve similar results [8, 9]. However, problems remain, including concerns about poor quality, cost, underdetection, radiation exposure, and overdiagnosis. Ongoing research is investigating ways to improve LDCT screening and evaluating the ability of biomarkers to improve risk and diagnosis with the aim of improving patients.

6.1.3 Role of Machine Learning in Medical Diagnostics

Cancer, known for its suffering and deaths, poses a serious threat to health, emphasizing the importance of early diagnosis and treatment. PET/CT scans are often used for early detection, staging, and treatment evaluation, especially in cancer. However, due to tumor heterogeneity and low image resolution, PET/CT imaging alone may not provide a good image of the tumor. Artificial intelligence (AI), particularly through ML, is increasingly being used in many areas, including lung cancer diagnosis and treatment [12]. AI involves using computers to test human intelligence and reasoning, leading to advances in science and technology [10, 11, 18]. Key areas of expertise include systems thinking, planning, case theory, and fuzzy systems. ML is a major branch of AI that enables machines to change human behavior by creating algorithms from big data and learning from experience.

Essentially, machines can "learn" from data (sometimes without human intervention) by creating programs and mathematical models and making high-level predictions or decisions about similar information. Generally speaking, the more data there is, the better the model will be, so data storage and processing capabilities are important for training ML models [15]. ML uses four main learning methods: reinforcement learning, supervised learning, unsupervised learning, and semi-supervised learning, each designed for a specific type of task.

K nearest neighbor (KNN), NB, LR, SVM, random forest (RF), decision tree (DT), backpropagation artificial neural network (BP-ANN), and adaptive boosting (AdaBoost), among others. The majority of these algorithms are classified as supervised learning algorithms. With the rapid advancement of science and technology, new research has emerged in ML: deep learning (DL), sample design, and sample delivery [16, 19]. Each step has different functions that are not explained below.

Some important terms in ML are frequently used and need to be explained. The training process is the data used to build the model, the validation process is used to tune the model's hyperparameters, and the testing process is used to test the model's ability to generalize to new data.

6.2 Machine Learning Techniques Used in Lung Cancer Detection

Cancer is a serious and deadly disease that kills approximately 422 people worldwide every day. Deadly because it is harder to detect than other diseases. The study of knowledge structures and cognitive processes is the foundation of ML, a subfield of AI. Developing models and algorithms that can learn from and adjust to large amounts of data is its main goal [25]. Using historical data and recognized trends, ML algorithms are able to evaluate this data and provide predictions and judgments. Human needs and relationships exist. ML algorithms may expand and forecast new, unseen data, and the model learns during training from a sample or historical data. AI, language processing, recommendation, picture and audio recognition, and self-driving cars are just a few of the numerous uses for ML. It has become an important tool for understanding, streamlining, and improving decision-making across businesses.

DL, a more advanced form of ML, excels at challenging tasks including item extraction, object identification, speech recognition, and other challenges in handling complex data. DL uses a multilayer deep neural network to identify and learn complex patterns in data and has shown great potential in many areas, often achieving remarkable results and some superhuman performances [28, 29].

The practice of using information from one job to enhance the performance of related tasks is known as learning through transfer (TL) in ML and DL. When there are specialized tools available for this purpose, TL can be quite beneficial. It has two main applications: as a framework for performance evaluation and for image dataset training.

In contrast, clustering involves combining several unique models to solve problems like classification. This ML technique improves prediction accuracy by combining the results of multiple models. Ensemble learning is also an important research focus on improving the performance of classification models [30, 31].

Numerous research studies have looked into various techniques for diagnosing cancer. Since 2019, the World Health Organization (WHO) has declared the coronavirus (COVID-19) to be a worldwide pandemic due to its alarming global spread. Currently, nucleic acid testing is the primary technique for identifying COVID-19, but it occasionally yields false-positive findings. Lung CT scans provide a more reliable method for screening and monitoring confirmed patients. Computer-aided diagnostic (CAD) technology can empower doctors by making faster and more accurate diagnoses. CAD systems use image fusion, medical imaging technology, and computer analysis to increase the accuracy and efficiency of diagnostic procedures [32, 33].

6.2.1 Lung Cancer Treatment Using CAD Method

The authors use four distinct datasets to describe a CAD based on U-Net and ResNet-34 structures. They employed a clinical segmentation metric called the Dice Similarity Coefficient (DSC), which calculates the overlap (from 0 to 1) between the actual and predicted segmentations, to assess the efficacy of their approach. A perfect match is indicated by a value of 1. According to the findings, the CAD system was accurate in recognizing and categorizing significant areas in medical pictures, as evidenced by its average DSC of over 0.93 across the four datasets. There are some limitations, especially when it comes to collaboration. However, the system achieved an F-score of 99.2% and an accuracy of over 99.3%. This study examines the systems added to our storage facility using two DL methods and a failure test using four performance metrics.

Multiple CT scans and the Gabor filter were used in the work of [13] to create a manual lung cancer screening method. Nine hundred of the 1,800 photographs in the database are of youngsters who have been diagnosed with lung cancer. Each image has a size of two hundred × two hundred pixels, and the information is taken from the IMBA Main Database. However, no precise measurements or findings were reported in this investigation. The highest accuracy of the CAD system is 99.61%, while the average accuracy is 99.42%. Additionally, it does exceptionally well on other parameters, as seen by its 99.76% recall, 99.88% accuracy, and 99.82% F-score, respectively.

6.2.2 CNN's Strategy for Preventing Lung Cancer

Ref. [14] introduced an updated convolutional neural network (CNN) model to estimate left ventricular volume using a multi-image fusion of MR images. In another study, [17] proposed an image fusion method using translationally invariant wavelets combined with stepwise principal component averaging (PCA). Experimental results show that this combination passes both visual and quantitative measurements. In addition, ref. [8] proposed a modified dictionary learning method for multi-image image fusion, which includes filtering out zero data and using multiple features to estimate the image section.

This effectively reduces the computational complexity while still providing good image quality. Similarly, [20] developed a LungNet deep CNN model with the aim of improving the accuracy of computer-aided diagnosis (CAD) of lung cancer. The model provides information from electronic devices that can be used as part of the Internet of Medical Things (MIoT) with CT scan images to improve the accuracy of diagnosis. LungNet uses a 22-layer CNN architecture to extract features from two sources and achieves 96.81% accuracy and a 3.35% false positive (FP) rate in five categories of lung cancer classification. It also achieved a 7.15% FP rate and a 91.6% accuracy rate in distinguishing stage 1 and stage 2 cancer. After training on 525,000 image sets, LungNet was run on the central server and showed promise in lung cancer diagnosis with minimum FP and high accuracy.

Another research suggested an artificial neural network (ANN) model for diagnosing cancer [21], which employs a number of symptoms to reach a conclusion. The model was trained and validated on lung cancer research data, and it achieved an accuracy of about 96.67% after completing more than 1,418,000 training sessions. However, the method discussed in this paper is more accurate, showing its advantages by achieving more than 99% with less training. Also, this method has a shorter execution time than the method in ref. [22]. The CAD system built in this study performed exceptionally well, with accuracy, recall, precision, and F-score reaching 99.42%, 99.76%, 99.88%, and 99.82%, respectively. To achieve these results, the researchers adapted and integrated two DL methods: VGG-19 and LSTM [35].

6.2.2.1 Diagnose Lung Cancer with DL and ML Methods

To enhance the performance of image categorization [23], a method is proposed that combines deep features generated by VGG19 DL models with unique methods created to get rid of technologies like Shi-Tomasi on detecting algorithms, ORB, SURF, and SIFT. These combined features are then used with various ML algorithms for classification. The results show that the RF classifier achieves the highest accuracy of 93.73% when combined with the features extracted by this method, outperforming other classifiers. This shows that using a combination of DL and traditional features is more effective and efficient than relying on only one extraction method.

A DL model based on the DarkNet-19 architecture was presented by the authors in [24] in order to produce picture clusters. This strategy chooses weak features from the patterns produced by the DarkNet-19 model by applying optimization approaches for balancing and efficient foraging. The optimal feature set is then produced by eliminating these weak characteristics. The pertinent characteristics produced by the two optimization techniques are categorized using the SVM approach. With a 99.69% accuracy rate and a 99.3% area under the curve (AUC) score, this classifier demonstrated outstanding performance. Additionally, with an F-test of 97.1%, the approach shows great accuracy, precision, recall, and F-test. The efficiency of integrating several optimization strategies and approaches to enhance dataset capabilities is demonstrated by this DL model. The indicators of performance that show how well the model can categorize pictures include the AUC, F-measure, accuracy, precision, and recall. The application of ML—more especially, forest-based models—to the early detection of cancer was examined in another research [26].

6.2.3 Lung Cancer Diagnosis by Combining Various Techniques

Ref. [27] developed a hybrid integrated feature extraction model for cancer diagnosis and tested it on the LC25000 lung dataset. The results showed that this hybrid model achieved 99.05% accuracy in lung cancer diagnosis, demonstrating its effectiveness in correct diagnosis. Furthermore, the model outperforms existing options, demonstrating its potential for clinical use. This illustrates how adaptive learning and integrated models might enhance lung cancer diagnosis by 90% and 89%, respectively, for DenseNet201. The accuracy percentage rose to 91% when these models were taken together, though. This demonstrates how altering the criteria can improve the diagnosis of lung cancer. Using feature extraction modules like DAISY and HOG, the Inception v3 model is included in the framework. The accuracy rate is as high as 99.60%, consistent with previous findings. These results demonstrate the potential of hybrid DL models as accurate cancer diagnosis techniques.

6.3 Machine Learning Approaches in Lung Cancer Detection

6.3.1 Traditional Machine Learning Approaches

6.3.1.1 Logistic Regression

The method utilized for LR to analyze data sets with independent variables to determine the probability. It creates a separation hyperplane between two data sets and provides data functions and vectors that represent the probability of a certain event based on different inputs. The technology is suitable for many areas, such as estimating disease risk and classifying data into different categories. For predicting applications, LR is a particularly helpful binary distribution technique. The logistic function, a sigmoid function (S-shaped curve) that depicts the weighted linear combination of characteristics for real values between 0 and 1, serves as the foundation for the methodology. Instead of just labeling an item, the model may assess the likelihood that it belongs to a specific category by interpreting these values as probabilities [36]. For example, one study developed a method that classified finger movements to control an upper-body prosthesis with 65% accuracy. Another study introduced a multiclass LR classifier to identify cardiac arrhythmias with 93.13% accuracy. LR is also used to predict the probability of failure in engineering. One study used partial least squares LR to develop a model that predicted business failure with 94.5% accuracy. LR is also used for hypothesis testing. For example, one study proposed a face recognition method using an LR classifier that achieved an accuracy of 96.84% when tested using the TFEID dataset [37]. LR is a mathematical modeling method for analyzing epidemiological data, particularly in the context of ML. The LR method can be executed in the following steps:

1. Use logical tools to calculate the values.
2. Determine the coefficients of the LR model.
3. Finally, the LR model is used for prediction. The logistic function is given below:

$$f(x) = \frac{L}{1 + e^{-K(x-x_0)}} \tag{6.1}$$

E = Euler number
x_0 = mean x value of sigmoid function
L = maximum value of the curve
K = degree of change of the curve.

Input value (x) to predict output value (y);
The equation of the LR model is as follows:

$$y = \frac{e^{bo+b1*x}}{1 + e^{bo+b1*x}} \tag{6.2}$$

With the training data, the log-likelihood function is maximized to estimate the LR parameters. An illustration of the use of LR to distinguish between two groups is shown in Figure 6.2.

6.3.1.2 SVMs, or Support Vector Machines

The best image-based ML systems are based on techniques such as SVM, linear regression, pruning trees, and KNN [34]. SVM is a popular method for prediction, regression, and classification tasks. It works by creating a boundary called a hyperplane that separates the incoming data into two different parts. A key advantage of SVM is its data-driven approach, which allows accurate classification without any prior assumptions, especially when the sample size is small. SVMs are widely used to classify biomarker data to predict and diagnose various diseases, including cancer, neurological diseases, and cardiovascular diseases [38]. Computational models

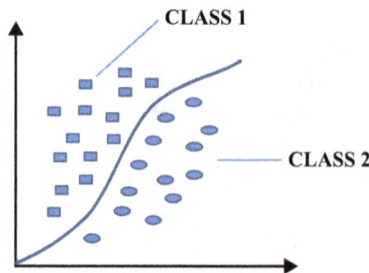

Figure 6.2 Distinguished classes of Logistic Regression

contain connecting units called neurons that respond to external stimuli. Neural networks operate in two phases: learning and testing. In the learning phase, the model deploys new ideas, and in the testing phase, the network processes input signals to produce output.

ANNs are useful in many areas of medicine, including breast cancer, cancer and other disease diagnosis and prediction, and drug analysis. The output results are a segment that depends on previous results. They use memory to store information about past results and allow them to make decisions about these points when connecting.

6.3.1.3 Decision Trees

A nonparametric learning method used for classification and regression is the decision tree. Roots, branches, stems, and leaves are part of the hierarchy. Decision tree learning uses a divide-and-conquer approach that uses greedy searches to determine the best split points in the tree. This segmentation process is repeated from top to bottom until all or most of the inputs are classified according to some label [39] (Figure 6.3).

Decision trees are a nonparametric supervised learning algorithm for classification and propagation. It has a hierarchical structure consisting of roots, branches, internodes, and leaves. Using greedy search to find the optimal distribution inside the tree, decision tree learning applies the divide and conquer strategy. Up until the majority of the items are assigned a single label, this segmentation procedure is repeated from top to bottom. The intricacy of the decision tree often influences how data points are categorized into homogenous groups. Small trees facilitate the use of transparent sheets where all data points are in a single group. However, as the tree grows, this purity becomes difficult to maintain and often results in insufficient information in the tree. This problem is called data fragmentation and can result in overfitting. Therefore, the tree decided to emphasize a small structure according to the principle of simplicity in Occam's razor, "no space should be added unless value is created." In short, no matter how simple the model, a decision tree should be

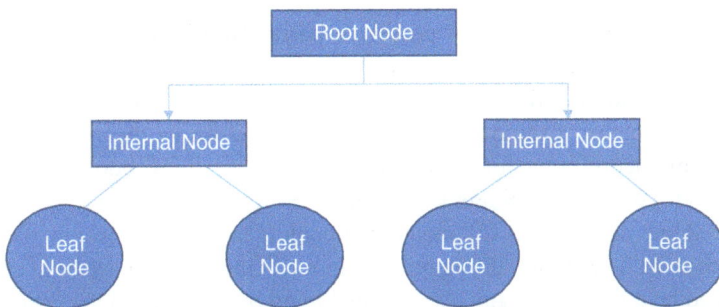

Figure 6.3   Tree Structure.

complex only when absolutely necessary [40, 41]. It involves removing branches that are different from unnecessary branches. The security of the model can be measured by competition. Another idea to verify the accuracy is to create an ensemble using the RF algorithm, which can improve the prediction accuracy, especially when the trees are not uniform.

6.3.1.4 Random Forests

In ML, the RF algorithm is a potent tree learning method. During training, it generates many decision trees. A random subset of the dataset is used to form each tree, and features are chosen at random from each partition. Because each tree is unique, this unpredictability lowers the chance of overfitting and enhances the forecast as a whole. Split the work and reinterpret its meaning by using voting. The data from several trees is used in this integrated decision-making approach to get accurate and effective outputs [42]. Because RFs can handle complicated data, cut down on overhead, and produce accurate predictions in a variety of applications, they are frequently employed in classification and regression.

6.3.1.5 K-Nearest Neighbors (k-NN)

KNN is a widely used classification algorithm in ML. It classifies objects by determining the closest points to the objects classified in training. Classification based on the closest points is called the nearest neighbor algorithm. Classification is essential for big data management, data science, and many ML applications. KNN is one of the oldest, simplest, and best model classification and regression algorithms. Many researchers have achieved significant improvements in accuracy by improving the KNN algorithm. This article aims to review the various advancements made by the KNN algorithm [43].

6.3.2 Deep Learning Approaches

6.3.2.1 Convolutional Neural Networks (CNNs)

CNNs are inspired by biological processes, particularly how the visual cortex of animals represents patterns of connections between neurons. The algorithm is particularly useful for multi-class problems and binary classification tasks, such as determining whether a tumor is present in a medical image. A typical CNN has several components: convolution layers, activation functions, pooling layers, and output layers. While a CNN uses weights during the convolution process to change the pixel values of the input CT image, the pooling layer performs downsampling. This leads to an iterative weighting process. In medicine, CNNs have been used successfully to help diagnose many diseases, including breast cancer, lung cancer, heart disease, and brain disease [44].

6.3.2.2 Recurrent Neural Networks (RNNs)

ANNs are designed to allow computers to process data efficiently, inspired by the structure of the human brain. This includes ML, especially DL, which uses networks or neurons that are organized in a hierarchical manner similar to the human brain. ANNs create an adaptive system that allows computers to learn from their mistakes and gradually improve their performance. Therefore, neural networks are designed to solve complex problems such as data collection and facial recognition with higher accuracy.

6.4 Applications and Performances for Lung Cancer Detection

Some of the first AI applications in this area focused on detecting lung nodules in X-ray and computed tomography (CT) scans, with performance levels comparable to or better than electron microscopy. The CNN-based algorithm applied to CT images for pulmonary nodule segmentation showed excellent spatial overlap with manual segmentation, even for weak and ground-glass nodules. Another important application of these features is the classification of lung nodules as malignant or benign, which can help narrow down CT scans to those that are suspicious.

Several algorithms have proven useful in predicting the risk of malignancy once nodules are detected. The use of AI in lung nodule analysis is particularly promising in the context of lung cancer diagnosis. They can help characterize tumors, especially by predicting histological subtypes and somatic alterations that may affect treatment. In addition, these tools, when combined with clinical data, can help predict patient outcomes. Despite these hopes, however, the clinical use of AI is still in its early stages due to challenges such as a lack of a wide range of published studies, poor performance, and insufficient data on how these tools affect radiologists' decisions and patient outcomes [45]. It is important for electronics scientists to participate in the evaluation of smart devices because these technologies can enhance their daily work and allow them to focus on more important work.

6.5 Challenges and Limitations

AI, especially through DL, is paving the way for progress in the evaluation of lung nodules and lung cancer. New equipment has been developed to support and enhance the work of radiologists, especially with the widespread use of CT cancer examinations worldwide. This tool is particularly useful due to the increasing workload of radiologists and the urgent need to identify more suspicious nodules; this can help reduce negativity and facilitate self-examination. It can also be useful for young radiologists with limited clinical experience. However, despite many publications focusing on DL in pulmonary nodule and lung cancer research, the clinical use of this technology has been delayed for several reasons. Heterogeneity makes it difficult to synthesize findings and support individual author claims. Differences in datasets, algorithm architectures, implementation models, and performance metrics make comparisons possible. Many studies lack external validation of independent data and often do not follow up on the work of radiologists, raising concerns about the generality and validity of publishing DL algorithms. The electronic AI checklist suggested by the authors can help readers deeply evaluate the research. Obstacles: The inner workings of these models are often opaque, often referred to as "black boxes," and lack a theoretical basis. Users need to have a clear understanding of how AI tools work in order to trust their implementation. An algorithm must demonstrate an additional advantage in terms of speed, performance, or cost, even if it makes a correct diagnosis compared to an electronic one. Finally, the impact of AI on radiologists' decision-making processes and the impact on patient care and outcomes are largely unknown.

6.6 Future Directions and Conclusion

The future of AI applications in lung cancer will focus on collaboration and strategy. First, given that AI is the foundation of data-driven technology, researchers can improve training by combining small data sets to recreate large data sets. However, management issues related to data sharing make this process difficult. State training, which allows sharing training without changing the raw material, is an important opportunity. In this way, models are trained separately in different hospitals, and only training models are sent to the central server, thus preventing direct access to data-sensitive paper.

The final sample was returned to the hospital. However, multiple integrations, including electronics, viruses, demographics, health information, and existing and emerging technologies, are coming voluntarily to raise lung cancer awareness. These different approaches can help researchers develop predictive models and support the concept of multidisciplinary omics, or "medical omics." Just as collaborative teams are important in managing lung cancer treatment, future research should also source information from multiple sources. Another important issue is the use of AI programs. Although early studies have shown good results in the use of AI for lung cancer, and some products have been approved by the FDA, their practical application in clinical practice is still limited. Factors such as user interface design, data analysis speed, AI applications, network bandwidth, and resource requirements for implementation pose challenges for real-world deployment. Significant advances in infrastructure will be needed before we can experience AI-powered healthcare.

References

1 Danjuma, K.J. Performance Evaluation of Machine Learning Algorithms in Post-operative Life Expectancy in the Lung Cancer Patients. Department of Computer Science, Modibbo Adama University of Technology, Yola, Adamawa State, Nigeria, 2015.

2 Karhan, Z.; Tunç, T. Lung Cancer Detection and Classification with Classification Algorithms. *IOSR Journal of Computer Engineering (IOSR-JCE)*, 2016, 18(6), 71–77.

3 Kaur, A.R. A Study of Detection of Lung Cancer Using Data Mining Classification Techniques. *International Journal of Advanced Research in Computer Science and Software Engineering*, 2013, 3.

4 Dwivedi, S.A.; Borse, R.P.; Yametkar, A.M. Lung Cancer Detection and Classification by Using Machine Learning & Multinomial Bayesian. *IOSR Journal of Electronics and Communication Engineering (IOSR-JECE)*, 2014, 9(1), 69–75.

5 Bawane, K. V.; Shinde, A. V. Diagnosis Support System for Lung Cancer Detection Using Artificial Intelligence. *International Journal of Innovative Research in Computer and Communication Engineering* 2018, 6(1).

6 Al-Absi, H.R.H.; Samir, B. B., Shaban, K. B.; Sulaiman, S. Computer Aided Diagonosis System Based on Machine Learning Techniques for Lung Cancer. *2012 International Conference on Computer and Information Science (ICCIS)*, Kuala Lumpeu, 2012, 295–300.

7 Kaur, S. Comparative Study Review on Lung Cancer Detection Using Neural Network and Clustering Algorithm. *International Journal of Advanced Research in Electronics and Communication Engineering (IJARECE)* 2015, 4(2).

8 Vinitha, D.; Gupta, D.; Khare, S. Exploration of Machine Learning Techniques for Cardiovascular Disease. *Applied Medical Informatics* 2015, 36, 23–32.

9 Sathyan, H., Panicker, J.V. Lung Nodule Classification Using Deep ConvNets on CT Images. *9th International Conference on Computing, Communication and Networking Technologies, ICCCNT 2018*, 2018.

10 Isaac, J.; Harikumar, S. Logistic Regression within DBMS. *Proceedings of the 2016 2nd International Conference on Contemporary Computing and Informatics, IC3I 20167918045*, pp. 661–666, 2016.

11 Siegel, R.L.; Miller, K.D.; Jemal, A. Cancer Statistics, 2020. *CA Cancer J. Clin.* 2020, 70, 7–30.

12 Sung, H.; Ferlay, J.; Siegel, R.L.; Laversanne, M.; Soerjomataram, I.; Jemal, A.; Bray, F. Global Cancer Statistics 2020: GLOBOCAN Estimates of Incidence and Mortality Worldwide for 36 Cancers in 185 Countries. *CA Cancer J. Clin.* 2021, 71, 209–249.

13 Cifci, M.A. SegChaNet: A Novel Model for Lung Cancer Segmentation in CT Scans. *Appl. Bionics Biomech.* 2022, 2022, 1139587.

14 Jakimovski, G.; Davcev, D. Using Double Convolution Neural Network for Lung Cancer Stage Detection. *Appl. Sci.* 2019, 9, 427.

15 Wang, J.;Wang, J.;Wen, Y.; Lu, H.; Niu, T.; Pan, J.; Qian, D. Pulmonary Nodule Detection in Volumetric Chest CT Scans Using CNNs-Based Nodule-Size-Adaptive Detection and Classification. *IEEE Access* 2019, 7, 46033–46044.

16 Wang, C.; Chen, D.; Hao, L.; Liu, X.; Zeng, Y.; Chen, J.; Zhang, G. Pulmonary Image Classification Based on Inception-v3 Transfer Learning Model. *IEEE Access* 2019, 7, 146533–146541.

17 Razzak, M.I.; Naz, S.; Zaib, A. Deep Learning for Medical Image Processing: Overview, Challenges and the Future. *Lect. Notes Comput. Vis. Biomech.* 2018, 26, 323–350.

18 Shao, J.; Wang, G.; Yi, L.; Wang, C.; Lan, T.; Xu, X.; Guo, J.; Deng, T.; Liu, D.; Chen, B.; et al. Deep Learning Empowers Lung Cancer Screening Based on Mobile Low-Dose Computed Tomography in Resource-Constrained Sites. *Front. Biosci. Landmark* 2022, 27, 212.

19 Wang, C.; Xu, X.; Shao, J.; Zhou, K.; Zhao, K.; He, Y.; Li, J.; Guo, J.; Yi, Z.; Li, W. Deep Learning to Predict EGFR Mutation and PD-L1 Expression Status in Non-Small-Cell Lung Cancer on Computed Tomography Images. *J. Oncol.* 2021, 2021, 5499385.

20 Li, R.; Xiao, C.; Huang, Y.; Hassan, H.; Huang, B. Deep Learning Applications in Computed Tomography Images for Pulmonary Nodule Detection and Diagnosis: A Review. *Diagnostics* 2022, 12, 298.

21 Lakshmanaprabu, S.K.; Mohanty, S.N.; Shankar, K.; Arunkumar, N.; Ramirez, G. Optimal Deep Learning Model for Classification of Lung Cancer on CT Images. *Future Gener. Comput. Syst.* 2019, 92, 374–382.

22 Lee, S.M.; Seo, J.B.; Yun, J.; Cho, Y.H.; Vogel-Claussen, J.; Schiebler, M.L.; Gefter, W.B.; van Beek, E.J.; Goo, J.M.; Lee, K.S.; et al. Deep Learning Applications in Chest Radiography and Computed Tomography. *J. Thorac. Imaging* 2019, 34, 75–85.

23 Deep Learning Applications in Chest Radiography and Computed Tomography. *J. Thorac. Imaging* 2019, 34, 75–85.

24 Bhatia, S.; Sinha, Y.; Goel, L. Lung Cancer Detection: A Deep Learning Approach. In *Soft Computing for Problem Solving: SocProS 2017*; Springer: Singapore, 2019; Volume 2, pp. 699–705.

25 Tian, P.; He, B.; Mu, W.; Liu, K.; Liu, L.; Zeng, H.; Liu, Y.; Jiang, L.; Zhou, P.; Huang, Z.; et al. Assessing PD-L1 Expression in Non-Small Cell Lung Cancer and Predicting Responses to Immune Checkpoint Inhibitors Using Deep Learning on Computed Tomography Images. *Theranostics* 2021, 11, 2098.

26 Ashraf, S.F.; Yin, K.; Meng, C.X.; Wang, Q.; Wang, Q.; Pu, J.; Dhupar, R. Predicting Benign, Preinvasive, and Invasive Lung Nodules on Computed Tomography Scans Using Machine Learning. *J. Thorac. Cardiovasc. Surg.* 2022, 163, 1496–1505.

27 Subramanian, R.R.; Mourya, R.N.; Reddy, V.P.T.; Reddy, B.N.; Amara, S. Lung Cancer Prediction Using Deep Learning Framework. *Int. J. Control. Autom.* 2020, 13, 154–160.

28 Vani, R.; Vaishnnave, M.P.; Premkumar, S.; Sarveshwaran, V.; Rangaraaj, V. Lung Cancer Disease Prediction with CT Scan and Histopathological Images Feature Analysis Using Deep Learning Techniques. *Results Eng.* 2023, 18, 101111.

29 Shalini, W.; Vigneshwari, S. A Novel Hybrid Deep Learning Method for Early Detection of Lung Cancer Using Neural Networks. *Healthc. Anal.* 2023, 3, 100195.

30 Abunajm, S.; Elsayed, N.; ElSayed, Z.; Ozer, M. Deep Learning Approach for Early-Stage Lung Cancer Detection. arXiv 2023, arXiv:2302.02456, 2023.

31 Deng, J.; Dong, W.; Socher, R.; Li, L.J.; Li, K.; Li, F.-F. ImageNet: A Large-Scale Hierarchical Image Database. In *Proceedings of the IEEE Conference on Computer Vision and Pattern Recognition (CVPR)*, Miami, FL, 20–25 June 2009; pp. 248–255.

32 Ye, Y.; Zhang, Y.; Yang, N.; Gao, Q.; Ding, X.; Kuang, X.; Bao, R.; Zhang, Z.; Sun, C.; Zhou, B.; et al. Profiling of Immune Features to Predict Immunotherapy Efficacy. *Innovation* 2022, 3, 100194.

33 Hao, T.; Kim, D.R.; Xie, X. Automated Pulmonary Nodule Detection Using 3D Deep Convolutional Neural Networks. In *Proceedings of the 2018 IEEE 15th International Symposium on Biomedical Imaging (ISBI 2018)*, Washington, DC, 4–7 April 2018; IEEE: New York.

34 Zaffino, P.; Marzullo, A.; Moccia, S.; Calimeri, F.; De Momi, E.; Bertucci, B.; Arcuri, P.P.; Spadea, M.F. An open-source COVID-19 CT Dataset with Automatic Lung Tissue Classification for Radiomics. *Bioengineering* 2021, 8, 26.

35 Prior, F.; Smith, K.; Sharma, A.; Kirby, J.; Tarbox, L.; Clark, K.; Bennett, W.; Nolan, T.; Freymann, J. The public cancer radiology imaging collections of the Cancer Imaging Archive. *Sci. Data* 2017, 4, 170124.

36 Zhang, G.; Yang, Z.; Jiang, S. Automatic Lung Tumor Segmentation from CT Images Using Improved 3D Densely Connected UNet. *Med. Biol. Eng. Comput.* 2022, 60, 3311–3323.

37 Gindi, A.M.; Al Attiatalla, T.A.; Sami, M.M. A Comparative Study for Comparing Two Feature Extraction Methods and Two Classifiers in Classification of Earlystage Lung Cancer Diagnosis of Chest x-Ray Images. *J. Am. Sci.* 2014, 10, 13–22.

38 Raghu, V.K.; Zhao, W.; Pu, J.; Leader, J.K.;Wang, R.; Herman, J.; Yuan, J.-M.; Benos, P.V.; Wilson, D.O. Feasibility of Lung Cancer Prediction from Low-Dose CT Scan and Smoking Factors Using Causal Models. *Thorax* 2019, 74, 643–649.

39 Risse, E.K.; Vooijs, G.P.; van Hof, M.A. Relationship between the Cellular Composition of Sputum and the Cytologic Diagnosis of Lung Cancer. *Acta Cytol.* 1987, 31, 170–176.

40 MacDougall, B.;Weinerman, B. The Value of Sputum Cytology. *J. Gen. Intern. Med.* 1992, 7, 11–13.

41 Kennedy, T.C.; Hirsch, F.R.; Miller, Y.E.; Prindiville, S.; Murphy, J.R.; Dempsey, E.; Proudfoot, S.; Bunn, P.A.; Franklin, W.A. A Randomized Study of Fluorescence Bronchoscopy versus White-Light Bronchoscopy for Early Detection of Lung Cancer in High Risk Patients. *Lung Cancer* 2000, 1(Suppl. S1), 244–245.

42 Toyoda, Y.; Nakayama, T.; Kusunoki, Y.; Iso, H.; Suzuki, T. Sensitivity and Specificity of Lung Cancer Screening Using Chest Low-Dose Computed Tomography. *Br. J. Cancer* 2008, 98, 1602–1607.

43 Hinton, G. Deep Learning—A Technology with the Potential to Transform Health Care. *JAMA* 2018, 320, 1101–1102.

44 LeCun, Y.; Bengio, Y.; Hinton, G. Deep Learning. *Nature* 2015, 521, 436–444.

45 Havaei, M.; Davy, A.; Warde-Farley, D.; Biard, A.; Courville, A.; Bengio, Y.; Pal, C.; Jodoin, P.-M.; Larochelle, H. Brain Segmentation with Deep Neural Networks. *Medical Image Analysis* 2017, 35, 18–31.

Chapter 7

A Review on AI Approaches for the Detection of Diabetic Retinopathy

Gayana J Kumar, Kavitha D N and Vedavathi N

7.1 Introduction

Diabetic Retinopathy (DR) is a vascular complication of diabetes observed for the first time by Eduard Jaeger in 1856. It is a dysfunction of the retinal blood vessels due to chronic hyperglycemia. It is identified that after 20 years of diabetes, 99% of patients have Type 1 DM and 60% of patients have Type 2 DM. From these statistics, we can say that it is more common in Type 1 DM, which is associated with insulin in the body because of the defect in producing insulin by beta cells of the pancreas. The World Health Organization (WHO) reported a rise in patients suffering from diabetes to 422 million in 2014. By 2025, the number of DR patients is expected to increase further [1]. DR is a common cause of blindness. Damage to the blood vessels in the eye's tissues is a key cause of DR [2]. Initial symptoms of an eye condition include floaters, complex color perception, and impaired vision. The retina is made up of blood vessels that provide nutrients to it [3]. Diabetes inhibits blood vessel function, preventing the retina from receiving an adequate blood supply. DR is a long-term micro-vascular disorder that produces capillary blockages and hemorrhages in the retina [4]. Glaucoma is a condition in the eyes caused by increased eye pressure that damages the optic nerve, which transmits information to

 DOI: 10.1201/9781003617013-7

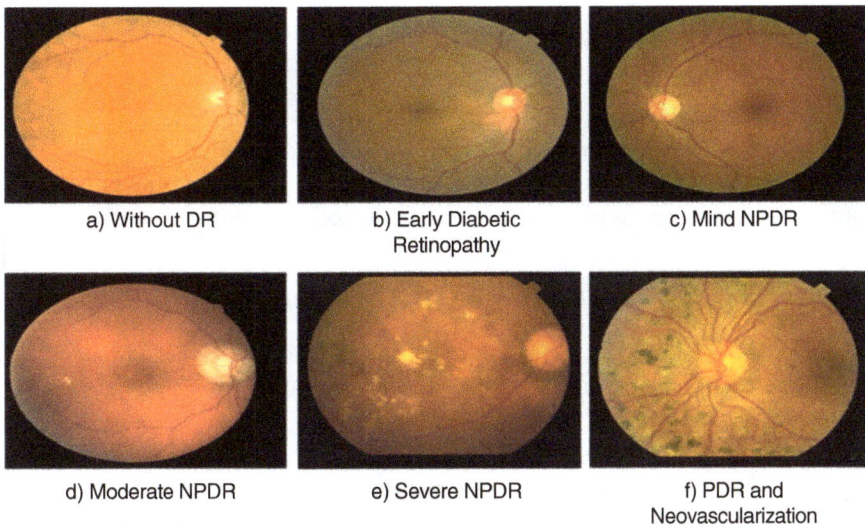

| a) Without DR | b) Early Diabetic Retinopathy | c) Mind NPDR |

| d) Moderate NPDR | e) Severe NPDR | f) PDR and Neovascularization |

Figure 7.1   Stages of DR [8].

the brain [5]. Early detection and treatment can prevent further progression and save many people from blindness. Diagnosing DR involves identifying specific retina lesions, including automated segmentation, blood vessel detection, soft and hard exudates, hemorrhages, and microaneurysms (MA) [6, 7]. The DR grading system is divided into two clusters: binary classification for diabetic retinas and multi-class classification for damaged retinas, ranging from healthy to proliferative. Figure 7.1 depicts the various stages of DR, indicating the development of MA [9]. In the middle stage, blood vessel bumps might lead to impaired vision. During the severe phase, blood vessels form abnormally and become fully crowded, which is possible. Segmenting retinal blood vessels in a picture can help provide the most effective treatment. Over the years, various technology-aided diagnosis techniques have been developed to detect and diagnose DR. The CAD for early diagnosis is a well-known and complicated challenge in medicine [10].

DR is a complication of diabetes that affects the eyes. It progresses through four stages and is categorized into two types: Nonproliferative Diabetic Retinopathy (NPDR) and Proliferative Diabetic Retinopathy (PDR). NPDR is considered the early stage of the disease, while PDR represents the more advanced stage.

7.1.1 Stage 1: Mild Nonproliferative Diabetic Retinopathy

In the initial stage of DR, known as Mild Nonproliferative DR, small areas of swelling, called MA, develop in the blood vessels of the retina. These MAs can cause a minor leakage of fluids into the retina, leading to swelling in the macula, the central part of the retina. Typically, this stage does not present any noticeable symptoms.

7.1.2 Stage 2: Moderate Nonproliferative Diabetic Retinopathy

As the condition progresses to moderate NPDR, the blood vessels in the retina swell further and begin to impede blood flow. This reduced blood flow can lead to a buildup of fluids and blood in the macula, causing vision to become blurry. The blockage of blood vessels means the retina is not receiving adequate nourishment.

7.1.3 Stage 3: Severe Nonproliferative Diabetic Retinopathy

In severe NPDR, a significant portion of the retinal blood vessels becomes blocked, severely restricting blood flow. This inadequate blood supply prompts the body to attempt to grow new blood vessels in the retina. However, these newly formed vessels are fragile and can cause further issues. They often lead to retinal swelling, which results in blurry vision, dark spots, and even patches of vision loss. If these vessels leak into the macula, it can cause sudden and potentially irreversible vision loss.

7.1.4 Stage 4: Proliferative Diabetic Retinopathy

PDR is the most advanced stage of DR. In this stage, new, weak blood vessels continue to grow within the retina. These vessels are prone to bleeding, which can lead to the formation of scar tissue inside the eye. The scar tissue can pull the retina away from the back of the eye, resulting in retinal detachment. This detachment can cause blurriness, a reduced field of vision, and even permanent blindness if not treated promptly.

The rest of the chapter is organized as follows: The related work is explained in Section 2. The research challenges and opportunities are discussed in Section 3. At last, the conclusion of this research work is summarized in Section 4.

7.2 Related Work

There are various approaches for detecting DR. Many automated models and solutions based on AI have been explored in recent years. This section presents some of the research work carried out in efficiently detecting the DR and various techniques for DR classification.

In the study titled "Vision Transformer Model for Predicting the Severity of Diabetic Retinopathy in Fundus Photography-Based Retina Images," the authors propose an adaptation of the Vision Transformer (ViT) model to automate the classification of DR. To correct imbalances in the dataset and improve training accuracy, the study uses six image augmentation techniques and picture normalization on top of the 1,842 high-resolution retinal images annotated by ophthalmologists found in the FGADR dataset. To reduce class imbalance, the dataset is divided into training

(80%), validation (10%), and testing (10%) sets using data balancing approaches. Pre-trained using ImageNet2012 and ImageNet21k, the ViT-Base and ViT-Large models are trained and verified; the ViT-Large model performs better when 32x32 patches are used. The study highlights several drawbacks despite its effectiveness, including dependency on a single dataset, the high computational demands of ViT models, and the requirement for high-quality annotated data. The outcomes demonstrate the potential of the ViT model in medical picture interpretation by indicating that it provides predictions that are more accurate than those of modern algorithms. In order to enhance model performance and confirm its application across various medical imaging datasets, the authors recommend conducting additional research [11].

The work by Alahmadi et al. [12] presents a unique deep learning model that leverages an attention strategy to use textural cues to improve the detection of DR. The preprocessing processes in the methodology include center cropping, bicubic interpolation for image scaling, and Graham's method-like enhancement to emphasize lesions and blood arteries. An inception encoder uses concurrent convolution processes to record multi-scale representations, which leads to more reliable feature extraction. The model breaks down features into two categories: style and content. Style deals with color and texture, while content is more concerned with structure and meaning. Two attention mechanisms are used: a Texture Attention Module that strengthens style-content associations and emphasizes high-frequency texture-related characteristics using the Laplacian pyramid approach and a Content Attention Module. The model has drawbacks despite its effectiveness, including the possibility of bias from training data, a rise in computational complexity, and the possibility of overfitting if the dataset is not sufficiently diverse. The study reveals that adding texture information greatly increases the accuracy of DR classification. The authors recommend that future research focus on data variability, computing effectiveness, and wider application to different medical imaging tasks [2].

In [13], the authors present a novel method that combines regression and classification tasks to improve precision in identifying the five stages of DR: no DR, mild DR, moderate DR, severe DR, and proliferative DR. The methodology makes use of the APTOS 2019 and EyePACS datasets, which contain 3,662 and 35,126 retinal pictures, respectively. Images are resized to 299x299 pixels, and various augmentation techniques are applied. The model architecture consists of a regression model for continuous severity scores and an SE-DenseNet-based classification model. The features of these models are integrated into a Multilayer Perceptron (MLP) for final classification. Stochastic gradient descent (SGD) is used in training for the classification model, and the Adam optimizer is used for the regression model. Regardless of its effectiveness, obstacles encompass imbalanced data, escalated computational requirements, and the possibility of overfitting. Using the APTOS and EyePACS datasets, the model demonstrated major improvements in classification accuracy, with weighted Kappa scores of 0.90 and 0.88, respectively. Subsequent investigations need to tackle data asymmetry, reduce computational complexity, and validate the model using additional datasets [13].

The paper by Kazi Ahnaf Alavee et al. proposes a hybrid strategy to enhance the early diagnosis of DR that combines explainable artificial intelligence (XAI) methods with deep learning (DL) models. In order to generate predictions that can be recognized, the approach involves collecting and preprocessing retinal fundus pictures, applying convolutional neural networks (CNNs) for early detection and classification, and combining XAI techniques such as Grad-CAM and LIME. Comprehensive datasets are used to train the DL models, while XAI is used to preserve interpretability. Criteria for evaluation include F1-score, accuracy, precision, recall, and interpretability scores. Robustness is ensured by cross-validation and different testing datasets. The study highlights that diagnostic accuracy and interpretability have improved, but there are still issues to be resolved. These include a more sophisticated system, possible trade-offs in performance, reliance on high-quality data, and significant computational resource requirements. The effective and broad clinical implementation of this approach, which provides increased diagnostic accuracy and clinician confidence in AI-based solutions for DR detection, depends on overcoming these challenges [14].

Zhentao Gao et al. explored the use of retinal fundus images to diagnose DR using deep neural networks (DNNs). To improve robustness, the approach involves collecting and preparing retinal images from medical databases using methods like augmentation, scaling, and normalization. To accurately identify and categorize DR stages, a customized DNN architecture is used for image classification. This architecture was trained on a large dataset of annotated retinal images. Metrics such as precision, recall, accuracy, and F1-score are used to assess the model's performance. To guarantee generalizability, cross-validation and testing on other datasets are also conducted. Regardless of its potential, the study highlights drawbacks such as dependency on abundant and high-quality data, difficulties in generalizing to new datasets with different characteristics, high computational resource requirements, and the interpretability of DNNs—which are frequently seen as black boxes in this field. According to the research, DNNs may significantly improve DR diagnosis, providing a valuable tool for early detection and treatment planning. However, for this technology to be broadly and effectively used in clinical settings, problems with data quality, model generalization, and resource needs must be resolved [15].

The paper by W.K. Wong, Filbert H. Juwono, and Catur Apriono studies an approach for the detection and grading of DR that combines feature-weighted Error-Correcting Output Codes (ECOC) ensemble with transfer learning. In order to improve model resilience, this method makes use of pre-trained CNNs that have been refined on retinal fundus images collected from medical databases. Preprocessing techniques, including normalization, augmentation, and scaling, are also used. While the feature-weighted ECOC ensemble increases the contribution of relevant features and enhances classification accuracy and robustness, simultaneous parameter optimization is carried out to fine-tune hyper-parameters. Accuracy, precision, recall, and F1-score are used to assess the performance of the model; cross-validation and testing on different datasets guarantee generalizability. Despite its effectiveness, the study highlights many drawbacks, including increased system complexity, dependence on diverse and high-quality data, significant computational requirements for resources, and generalization to previously untested datasets. The research results show that the hybrid technique can greatly increase the accuracy of grading and DR detection; nonetheless, resolving these issues is essential for wider clinical implementation [16].

In a survey by Mohammad Z. Atwany, Abdulwahab H. Sahyoun, and Mohammad Yaqub, the authors review deep learning approaches for classifying DR. The research addresses the importance of the quality of retinal fundus images as well as standard preprocessing techniques, including scaling, augmentation, and normalization. CNNs for feature extraction and classification, transfer learning using pre-trained models such as those on ImageNet, and ensemble techniques for increased accuracy and robustness are just a few of the deep learning architectures included in the survey. This work also addresses optimization and training strategies, emphasizing the application of different learning rates, loss functions, and regularization techniques. Metrics like F1-score, AUC-ROC, recall, accuracy, and precision are used to evaluate models. The survey highlights that although deep learning holds great potential for DR classification, there are several obstacles to overcome. These include the requirement for well-labeled data, the necessity to generalize to different datasets, the need for significant computational resources, and the interpretability of models. The study comes to the conclusion that although sophisticated approaches such as ensemble methods and transfer learning exhibit promise, more investigation is required to tackle these issues and enhance the precision, resilience, and clinical acceptability of DR classification models [17].

The paper by Fahman Saeed et al. explored how adaptively fine-tuning pre-trained CNNs can improve the detection of DR. The study utilizes preprocessing techniques such as normalization, augmentation, and scaling to prepare the data before using retinal fundus images from several medical databases. The process involves improving performance for DR detection by fine-tuning pre-trained models like VGG, ResNet, or Inception using the DR dataset and changing hyperparameters. To avoid overfitting, the models are iteratively trained through the use of batch normalization and dropout. Performance is assessed using standard metrics, while cross-validation is used to guarantee robustness. Although this approach shows promise in increasing the accuracy of DR diagnosis, there are still issues to be resolved, such as the need for balanced and high-quality data, challenges with generalizing to different datasets, high computational needs, and restricted interpretability of the model. The study concludes that adaptive CNN fine-tuning can improve automated DR diagnosis; however, in order to achieve wider clinical use and better patient outcomes, these issues must be addressed [18].

The research work [19] provides an approach for automatically identifying retinal lesions symptomatic of DR using image processing and machine learning. The image dataset of the retinal fundus is preprocessed, enhanced to highlight lesions, and resized for uniformity as part of the procedure. Lesion identification employs methods such as morphological operations, thresholding, and edge detection to identify MA, hemorrhages, exudates, and cotton wool spots. To classify lesions and establish DR phases, machine learning models such as support vector machines, decision trees, and random forests are trained using features that are extracted, including shape, size, color, and texture. To maximize performance, the models are trained using labeled datasets, hyperparameter tuning, and cross-validation. However, the quantity and quality of training data, the variety of lesion patterns, the demands on computational resources, and the interpretability of the model pose challenges to the effectiveness of the system. Despite these challenges, the work highlights the need to resolve data- and model-related concerns to improve clinical applicability and indicates promise in early DR diagnosis [19].

The authors in [20] propose an advanced method for improving the detection of DR using an ensemble of deep learning models. The approach involves utilizing fundus cameras to capture retinal images, which are then preprocessed using techniques like scaling, normalization, and Contrast Limited Adaptive Histogram Equalization (CLAHE) to improve image quality. DR characteristics are identified by independently training several CNN architectures, such as ResNet, DenseNet, and Inception, on these images. To create a reliable prediction system, the outputs of several models are then merged using ensemble methods including stacking, averaging, and voting. The ensemble model's generalizability is ensured through cross-validation, and it is assessed using accuracy, precision, recall, F1-score, and AUC-ROC. The ensemble approach has advantages over other approaches in terms of accuracy and robustness, but it also has drawbacks. These include increased computational complexity, dependence on diverse and high-quality data, concerns with clinical integration and maintenance, and interpretability issues. Although there is still room for improvement in DR identification with this ensemble method, more study is required to solve these issues and increase its usefulness in clinical situations [20].

The research by Anning Pan, Jingzong Yang et al. proposes the use of deep learning to monitor and detect temporal changes in DR lesions, allowing for timely intervention and treatment adjustments to avoid severe vision loss in diabetic patients. To improve lesion visibility, preprocessing techniques such as scaling, normalization, and CLAHE are used for retinal images that are obtained at various intervals. The images are analyzed using a CNN, which is trained on a dataset labeled with the presence and severity of DR lesions. The CNN is intended to identify and measure changes in lesions by comparing image pairs or sequences. In order to categorize changes as either no change, improvement, or worsening, the model evaluates spatial and intensity differences. Accuracy, sensitivity, specificity, and AUC-ROC are used to evaluate performance; cross-validation is used to ensure robustness. Although improved DR monitoring may be possible, there are a number of challenges to overcome, such as the need for diverse and high-quality data, substantial processing demands, retinal picture variability, and the interpretability of deep learning models. The study highlights the potential of deep learning in disaster recovery and recommends that future research concentrate on resolving these issues to enhance model interpretability, computational efficiency, and data quality for clinical integration [21].

In [22], the generation of artificial retinal images for DR detection and analysis using Generative Adversarial Networks (GANs) is explored, addressing issues with real-world dataset scarcity and imbalance. This study uses conditional GANs (cGANs) to produce synthetic visuals conditioned on particular types and stages of DR. A generator network creates realistic images, and a discriminator network distinguishes between actual and synthetic images. Actual retinal images with annotated DR lesions are preprocessed and utilized to train the GAN. As evaluated by quantitative criteria such as Fréchet Inception Distance (FID) and Inception Score (IS) as well as visual examination, the synthetic images are of greater quality after the adversarial training. By adding synthetic images to real datasets, machine learning models can be trained with greater diversity and balance. The study shows great promise despite several challenges, including the possibility of a quality mismatch between synthetic and real images, the computational intensity of training GANs, the risks of overfitting to synthetic data, and the subjective nature of evaluating synthetic images. The method can increase the DR diagnostic systems' robustness and accuracy, indicating that future studies should concentrate on improving the quality of synthetic images, streamlining the training procedure, and successfully incorporating synthetic data into clinical practice [22].

The study by Chu-Hui Lee and Yi-Hsuan Ke analyzes the classification of retinal fundus images for the purpose of detecting and grading DR using deep learning, specifically CNNs. For consistency and quality enhancement, preprocessing techniques such as scaling, normalization, and CLAHE are used for retinal images, which represent different stages of DR. The CNNs are trained on labeled datasets using architectures like ResNet, VGG, or Inception to identify and extract characteristics like MA, hemorrhages, and exudates that are suggestive of DR. The model uses cross-validation for robustness and classifies images into DR severity categories. Performance is assessed using measures such as accuracy, sensitivity, specificity, precision, recall, F1-score, and AUC-ROC. The research addresses challenges such as high computational requirements, variability in retinal images, data dependency, and the interpretability of deep learning models despite the possibility of early DR detection and improved patient outcomes. To further integrate these systems into clinical practice, future research should focus on improving model interpretability, computational efficiency, and data quality [23].

Mohammad Shorfuzzaman et al. addressed how to improve the grading of DR from retinal fundus images by integrating explainability into an ensemble of deep learning models. Using methods like scaling, normalization, and CLAHE for quality improvement, the methodology involves collecting and preprocessing retinal images. The outputs of multiple CNN architectures, such as ResNet, Inception, and DenseNet, are combined using ensemble techniques like voting, averaging, and stacking after they have been trained independently. To enhance interpretability, interpretable AI techniques such as Grad-CAM and LIME are integrated. These techniques provide saliency maps and heatmaps that emphasize significant areas of the image. The study demonstrates that explainable ensemble models have the ability to deliver accurate and interpretable DR despite their increasing complexity, computational costs, and dependency on high-quality data. This could lead to improved trust and acceptance of these models in clinical settings. Future studies should focus on enhancing data quality, facilitating a smooth integration into clinical workflows, and optimizing the trade-off between interpretability and accuracy [24].

The research work in [25] explores a deep learning system designed to identify DR in actual clinical settings—specifically, eye clinics in Thailand—that is put into practice and evaluated. The study, which is being carried out by researchers from Rajavithi Hospital and Google Health, focuses on interactions between patients, healthcare practitioners, and the AI system to evaluate the system's effectiveness from a human-centered perspective. Retinal image analysis for symptoms of DR was facilitated by the integration of a deep learning system into clinical procedures, which enabled immediate feedback. Data was collected using a combination of qualitative insights from patient and healthcare provider questionnaires and interviews, as well as quantitative indicators like the AI system's sensitivity and accuracy. Usability, workflow integration, user pleasure, and trust were important evaluation criteria. Initial integration issues with present workflows, healthcare providers' concerns about AI's dependability in comparison to clinical judgment, technical restrictions on image quality, and patient reactions to AI's involvement in diagnosis were among the challenges noted. In spite of these obstacles, the study came to the conclusion that using AI for DR detection can improve clinical practice diagnostic efficiency and accuracy. This research also emphasized the significance of providing healthcare providers with proper training, being open and honest in communication to build trust, and making sure AI complements rather than replaces human expertise. To optimize clinical utility and acceptance, this human-centered approach emphasizes how important it is to match AI implementations with healthcare professional needs and patient expectations [25].

The research work [26] explores a big data analytics technique for early DR detection within the Hadoop framework. The study focuses on managing large data sets made up of retinal images and related medical records by utilizing Hadoop's scalability and distributed computing capabilities. Key stages involve collecting data from various healthcare sources, standardizing datasets through preprocessing, and utilizing Hadoop components like HDFS and MapReduce to handle data efficiently. Features essential for diagnosing DR are extracted from images using image processing techniques, including segmentation and pattern recognition. These features are then examined by machine learning algorithms that have been trained on labeled datasets. Hadoop's big data analytics feature helps to find patterns that are useful for early disaster recovery identification. Despite Hadoop's scalability, challenges include inconsistent data quality that affects feature extraction accuracy, computational complexity, and the requirement for robust model generalization across different datasets. Overcoming adaptation barriers and guaranteeing smooth compatibility with existing healthcare systems are essential for integrating Hadoop-based technologies into clinical operations. The study highlights the potential of Hadoop in improving healthcare outcomes through sophisticated data analytics for early chronic disease detection, despite certain limitations. This research work also emphasizes the necessity of resolving technical and integration challenges for deployment in clinical settings [26].

The research work titled "Dual Branch Deep Learning Network for Detection and Stage Grading of Diabetic Retinopathy" will detect and grade the stages of DR; the research presents a novel deep learning architecture. The study begins with a large collection of retinal images that span several stages of deep learning. These images are preprocessed to eliminate noise, standardize resolution, and equalize intensity levels. The proposed dual-branch network consists of two specialized components: the first branch classifies images into distinct DR stages based on retrieved features, while the second branch concentrates on DR detection utilizing CNNs for feature extraction. During training, model parameters are optimized using methods like backpropagation, and model performance is evaluated using metrics like accuracy, sensitivity, and precision. By comparing the dual branch network with existing techniques, the study highlights cross-validation's robustness and generalizability. However, there are challenges in the way of clinical use, such as computational complexity, potential data imbalances that could affect model bias, and the interpretability of complex deep learning architectures. Despite these challenges, the dual branch network shows significant improvements in the accuracy of DR diagnosis, indicating that, with additional validation and tuning in clinical settings, it may improve the management of DR [27].

The research work titled "Smart Detection and Diagnosis of Diabetic Retinopathy using Bat-based Feature Selection Algorithm and Deep Forest Technique" presents a novel approach to improve the accuracy and efficiency of DR detection. The study utilizes an ensemble learning framework called deep forest for classification tasks and the bat algorithm for feature selection. The method seeks to enhance diagnostic results by utilizing deep forest models to identify DR severity levels and the bat algorithm's ability to retrieve discriminative characteristics from retinal images. To guarantee consistent input data quality, retinal images must be collected and preprocessed as part of the dataset preparation procedure. The model's performance is evaluated using metrics like accuracy and sensitivity, and cross-validation is taken into account to determine the model's generalizability. However, for wider clinical acceptance, challenges like computational complexity—especially in the feature selection and training phases—as well as concerns about the interpretability of the model and dataset representativeness must be resolved. The study emphasizes how cutting-edge feature selection techniques and advanced algorithms like deep forest can be combined to improve early DR detection and management practices [28].

A research work titled "Diabetic Retinopathy Detection Using Developed Hybrid Cascaded Multi-Scale DCNN with Hybrid Heuristic Strategy" presents an advanced methodology that uses heuristic optimization and deep learning to detect DR. The research suggests a hybrid cascaded multi-scale deep convolutional neural network (DCNN) architecture that is intended to improve sensitivity in identifying abnormalities linked to DR at different retinal image resolutions. This unique approach optimizes model parameters and increases classification accuracy by integrating a hybrid heuristic strategy that may involve simulated annealing or genetic algorithms. To ensure consistency and quality, preprocessing and collection of retinal images are part of the dataset preparation procedure. Metrics like accuracy and sensitivity are used in model evaluation and training, and cross-validation is used to guarantee robustness. However, challenges like the computational cost of implementing models and fine-tuning their parameters, together with concerns about the interpretability of complex deep learning architectures, point to areas that require focus before deep learning becomes widely used in clinical settings. The study emphasizes how early DR detection and management approaches can be advanced by combining advanced deep learning frameworks with heuristic strategies [29].

The study titled "Optimizing Diabetic Retinopathy Detection with Inception-V4 and Dynamic Version of Snow Leopard Optimization Algorithm" presents a novel approach that makes use of cutting-edge deep learning and optimization approaches to identify DR. The study uses the powerful Inception-V4 deep CNN, which is well-known for performing effectively in image classification applications because it has numerous inception modules which facilitate robust feature extraction at different resolutions and scales. A dynamic version of the Snow Leopard Optimization Algorithm (SLOA) is presented in order to improve the model's performance further. Through dynamic adjustments to exploration and exploitation techniques throughout the optimization process, this metaheuristic optimization technique improves both the speed of convergence and the quality of the solution. Preprocessing retinal images with annotations for different degrees of DR severity, such as noise reduction, augmentation, and normalization, is part of the dataset preparation process. The dynamic SLOA is used in the Inception-V4 model's training to optimize parameters with the goal of reducing classification errors and enhancing the model's discriminatory performance across a range of DR severity levels. Cross-validation ensures robustness and generalizability, while evaluation criteria including accuracy, sensitivity, specificity, and area under the ROC curve assess model performance. The appropriate management of computational complexity, efficient parameter optimization, and the interpretability of deep learning models provide challenges that must be addressed for clinical adoption and comprehension. While stressing the need for more validation and improvement to enhance real-world applicability, the study highlights the potential of combining cutting-edge deep learning architectures with adaptive optimization techniques to strengthen DR detection capabilities [30].

The research work titled "Automatic Detection and Monitoring of Diabetic Retinopathy Using Efficient Convolutional Neural Networks and Contrast Limited Adaptive Histogram Equalization" explores the use of CNNs in conjunction with CLAHE to detect and monitor DR automatically. By emphasizing important features including MA, hemorrhages, and exudates, CLAHE improves the contrast of retinal images and increases the accuracy of detection. Using a labeled dataset of retinal images, an effective CNN architecture with various convolutional, pooling, and fully connected layers is trained, allowing for the classification of DR severity and the tracking of disease progression. Challenges include dependence on the quantity as well as quality of training data, computational intensity, variability in retinal images due to different conditions and equipment, and the interpretability of CNNs in clinical situations, despite the system's high accuracy and durability. Although future research should concentrate on boosting model interpretability, maximizing computational efficiency, and improving data quality, the combination of CNNs with CLAHE shows promise in early DR diagnosis, suggesting potential for preventing vision loss in diabetic patients [31].

In [32], authors explored how AI might improve teleophthalmology's ability to diagnose DR. Fundus cameras are used in the system to capture retinal images, which are then preprocessed through stages including scaling and normalization. Contrast Limited Adaptive CLAHE is one technique used to improve image quality. To determine the extremity of DR, a CNN is put to use for feature extraction and classification. The CNN has been trained on a labeled dataset. The AI model supports remote diagnosis and monitoring by being integrated into a teleophthalmology platform with a user-friendly interface that allows medical professionals to upload images, view results, and access patient records. Metrics like accuracy and AUC-ROC are used to verify the model's performance against expert diagnosis. Data dependence, technological infrastructure, ethical and legal issues, and the requirement for user training are some of the challenges. Despite these challenges, the AI-based teleophthalmology application has significant potential to improve the accessibility and accuracy of DR detection, especially in areas with limited resources. However, more work is required to address existing limitations, expand datasets, and perform ample clinical trials for additional validation [32].

The research work by Zhitao Xiao et al., a deep learning framework designed for the classification of DR, is an important advancement in medical image analysis. To improve feature extraction and classification accuracy, SE-MIDNet makes use of multi-scale inception modules and squeeze-and-excitation (SE) blocks. The architecture of the network consists of inception modules to record a wide variety of features from smaller details to wider patterns and SE blocks to adjust channel-wise feature responses, emphasizing important elements in retinal images. To improve the adaptability of the model, data preprocessing includes normalization and augmentation methods, including rotation, flipping, and scaling. The Adam optimizer and a cross-entropy loss function are used in the training phase, along with regularization strategies like data augmentation and dropout to avoid overfitting. The model has significant drawbacks in terms of complexity and dependency on high-quality, diverse data, despite its excellent classification accuracy, sensitivity, and specificity for DR phases. Furthermore, SE-MIDNet's interpretability continues to be a problem. Subsequent studies should focus on improving interpretability and optimizing the design for quicker training. In general, SE-MIDNet presents a viable instrument for the prompt identification and treatment strategizing of DR, which may enhance patient results [33].

The study [34] explores the use of fundus photography for early detection of DR through the implementation of EfficientNet, a cutting-edge deep learning model. EfficientNet is a good choice for medical image classification tasks because of its ability to balance computational efficiency and accuracy, as well as its ability to scale over depth, width, and resolution. The methodology consists of applying transfer learning by fine-tuning EfficientNet pre-trained on ImageNet and preprocessing several kinds of fundus photographs via normalization and augmentation. To improve efficiency and avoid overfitting, the model is improved with the Adam optimizer utilizing a cross-entropy loss function with early halting and learning rate scheduling. Evaluation criteria that show the model's strong performance and validate its effectiveness in DR detection include accuracy, precision, recall, F1 score, and AUC-ROC. Although the results are reassuring, there are still challenges with model interpretability, computing resource requirements, and reliance on high-quality data. Subsequent investigations seek to strengthen the interpretability of the model, maximize training effectiveness, and expand the dataset's diversity. EfficientNet integration has the potential to greatly enhance patient outcomes and early DR detection in clinical workflows [34].

The authors, Md Sazzad Hossen et al., proposed an automated deep CNN model that employs retinal image categorization to detect DR early. The CNN architecture uses different multiple layers like convolutional layers, pooling layers, fully connected layers, and an output layer for classification to automatically extract features from retinal pictures. To ensure an accurate evaluation, an extensive set of labeled retinal images is divided into test, validation, and training sets. To increase the model's robustness, preprocessing methods, including normalization, scaling, and augmentation (including rotation and flipping), are used. The model is optimized with the Adam optimizer after being trained with a cross-entropy loss function. Batch normalization and dropout are used for regularization and to avoid overfitting. Despite its excellent performance, the model has limitations. The model was found to be complex; it has a high threshold for training computational resources and also interpretability issues and sensitivity to both the quality and quantity of data. These limitations highlight the need for more research to improve generalizability by diversifying datasets, optimizing training efficiency, and improving model interpretability. Improving patient outcomes and DR diagnosis through the use of this automated approach in clinical practice is a promising development [35].

The review titled "Diabetic Retinopathy Detection through Generative AI Techniques," examines the use of generative artificial intelligence (AI) techniques for the diagnosis of DR. The study classifies generative AI techniques, namely GANs and variational autoencoders (VAEs), and evaluates their efficacy using standard metrics—accuracy, sensitivity, and specificity. It does this by conducting a thorough literature review across databases like IEEE Xplore and PubMed. While the review emphasizes benefits like data augmentation and feature enhancement, it also highlights drawbacks such as model complexity and problems with the interpretability of generated images. Case studies highlight the potential of these strategies to enhance early diagnosis and management of DR by illuminating their practical application. To improve the robustness and clinical applicability of generative AI-driven DR detection systems, the review ends by outlining future research directions and arguing for developments in transfer learning and multimodal data fusion. This will yield penetrating information to researchers and healthcare professionals alike [36].

7.3 Research Challenges and Opportunities

Current AI approaches for detecting DR face several significant gaps that must be handled to improve their efficacy and real-time application. One major challenge is the imbalance in existing datasets [11], particularly the underrepresentation of severe DR cases. Balanced datasets from diabetes-prone regions such as India are crucial for developing robust models that generalize well across diverse populations. Furthermore, there is a need to establish platforms for real-time image submissions to facilitate swift disease decision-making in clinical settings. This can be achieved by developing user-friendly, easily deployable smartphone apps that allow for immediate processing and diagnosis, especially in resource-limited areas [14]. Ensuring the robustness of these platforms is essential to improve disease identification and management in medical imaging.

In addition to dataset issues, it is important to enhance transfer learning models and hybrid methods that blend deep learning with traditional image processing techniques. Existing transfer learning models require fine-tuning to improve accuracy and efficiency, especially for different stages of DR. Hybrid approaches show improvement but need more extensive research to validate their effectiveness in preprocessing and segmenting fundus images. Incorporating DR-related symptoms for multi-label classification and utilizing low-complexity CNNs can ease computational load at the same time as maintaining high prediction performance. Moreover, improving image preprocessing and segmentation algorithms can significantly enhance the quality of input images and the accuracy of diagnosis. Focusing on these areas will bridge the current gaps and lead to more reliable and accessible AI- and ML-based solutions for DR detection and classification.

7.4 Conclusion

This research work discussed the various approaches that are currently known and have shown better performance in the detection of DR. We also cited different methodologies available through extensive literature review. Based on the survey, it is observed that there exists a potential rationale for the early screening of DR using

AI techniques. Addressing the state-of-the-art AI, particularly deep learning approaches for DR detection, is essential for enhancing accuracy, efficiency, and real-time applicability. By creating balanced datasets, improving transfer learning models, and optimizing hybrid methods, the robustness of these systems can be significantly improved. Further research into image preprocessing and segmentation, as well as incorporating multi-label classification, will lead to more reliable and accessible diagnostic tools. These advancements will ultimately improve early detection and management of DR, particularly in resource-limited settings.

References

[1] Khanapur, S. & Patil, L. (2023). "A Study on Diabetic Retinopathy using Deep Learning Algorithms." *2023 International Conference on Integrated Intelligence and Communication Systems (ICIICS)*, Kalaburagi, India, 1–5, doi: 10.1109/ICIICS59993. 2023.10421731

[2] Farag, M. M., Fouad, M., & Abdel-Hamid, A. T. (2022). "Automatic Severity Classification of Diabetic Retinopathy Based on DenseNet and Convolutional Block Attention Module." *IEEE Access*, 10, 38299–38308, doi: 10.1109/ACCESS. 2022.3165193

[3] Nawaz, F., Ramzan, M., Mehmood, K., Khan, H.U., Khan, S.H., & Bhutta, M.R. (2020). "Early Detection of Diabetic Retinopathy Using Machine Intelligence through Deep Transfer and Representational Learning." *Comput. Mater. Contin.*, 66(2), 1631–1645, https://doi.org/10.32604/cmc.2020.012887

[4] Bengani, Shaleen, Angel Arul Jothi, J., & Vadivel, S. (2021). "Automatic Segmentation of Optic Disc in Retinal Fundus Images Using Semi-Supervised Deep Learning." *Multimedia Tools and Applications*, 80(3), 3443–3468, https://doi.org/10.1007/s11042-020-09778-6

[5] Alice, K., Deepa, N., Devi, T., BeenaRani, B.B., Bharatha Devi, N., & Nagaraju, V. (2023). "Effect of Multi Filters in Glucoma Detection Using Random Forest Classifier." *Measurement: Sensors*, 25, 100566, https://doi.org/10.1016/j.measen. 2022.100566

[6] Saeed, Fahman, Hussain, Muhammad, & Aboalsamh, Hatim. (2021). "Automatic Diabetic Retinopathy Diagnosis Using Adaptive Fine-Tuned Convolutional Neural Network." *IEEE Access*, 1, 10.1109/ACCESS.2021.3065273

[7] Qureshi, Imran, Ma, Jun, & Abbas, Qaisar (2021). "Diabetic Retinopathy Detection and Stage Classification in Eye Fundus Images Using Active Deep Learning." *Multimedia Tools and Applications*, 80(8), 11691–11721, https://doi.org/10.1007/s11042-020-10238-4

[8] Bidwai, Pooja, Gite, Shilpa, Pahuja, Kishore, & Kotecha, Ketan. (2022). A Systematic Literature Review on Diabetic Retinopathy Using an Artificial Intelligence Approach. *Big Data and Cognitive Computing*, 6(4), 152, https://doi.org/10.3390/bdcc6040152

[9] Sungheetha, Akey & Rajendran, Rajesh Sharma. (2021). Design an Early Detection and Classification for Diabetic Retinopathy by Deep Feature Extraction based Convolution Neural Network. *Journal of Trends in Computer Science and Smart Technology*, 3, 81–94, 10.36548/jtcsst.2021.2.002

[10] Vinayaki, V.D. & Kalaiselvi, R.. (2022). Multithreshold, Image Segmentation Technique Using Remora Optimization Algorithm for Diabetic Retinopathy Detection from Fundus Images. *Neural Processing Letters*, 54(3), 2363–2384, doi: 10.1007/s11063-021-10734-0. Epub 2022 Jan 24. PMID: 35095328; PMCID: PMC8784591.

[11] Nazih, Waleed, Aseeri, Ahmad, Youssef Atallah, Osama, & El-Sappagh, Shaker. (2023). "Vision Transformer Model for Predicting the Severity of Diabetic Retinopathy in Fundus Photography-Based Retina Image." *IEEE Access*, 11, 117546–117561, doi:10.1109/ACCESS.2023.3326528

[12] Alahmadi, Mohammad. (2022). "Texture Attention Network for Diabetic Retinopathy Classification." *IEEE Access*, 10, 55522–55532, doi:10.1109/ACCESS.2022.3177651

[13] Majumder, Sharmin & Kehtarnavaz, Nasser. (2021). Multitasking Deep Learning Model for Detection of Five Stages of Diabetic Retinopathy. *IEEE Access*, 9, 123220–123230, doi: 10.1109/ACCESS.2021.3109240

[14] Alavee, K.A., Hasan, M., Zillanee, A.H., Mostakim, M., Uddin, J., Alvarado, E.S., Diez, I.D.L.T., Ashraf, I., & Samad, M.A. (2024). "Enhancing Early Detection of Diabetic Retinopathy through the Integration of Deep Learning Models and Explainable Artificial Intelligence." *IEEE Access*, 12, 73950–73969, https://doi.org/10.1109/ACCESS.2024.3405570

[15] Gao, Zhentao, Li, Jie, Guo, Jixiang, Chen, Yuanyuan, Yi, Zhang, & Zhong, Jie. (2018). "Diagnosis of Diabetic Retinopathy Using Deep Neural Networks." *IEEE Access*, 7, 3360–3370, doi:10.1109/ACCESS.2018.2888639

[16] Wong, W. K., Juwono, F. H., & Apriono, C., "Diabetic Retinopathy Detection and Grading: A Transfer Learning Approach Using Simultaneous Parameter Optimization and Feature-Weighted ECOC Ensemble." *IEEE Access*, 11, 83004–83016, 2023. doi:10.1109/ACCESS.2023.3301618

[17] Atwany, Mohammad, Sahyoun, Abdulwahab, & Yaqub, Mohammad. (2022). "Deep Learning Techniques for Diabetic Retinopathy Classification: A Survey." *IEEE Access*, 10, 28642–28655, doi: 10.1109/ACCESS.2022.3157632

[18] Saeed, Fahman, Hussain, Muhammad, & Aboalsamh, Hatim. (2021). "Automatic Diabetic Retinopathy Diagnosis Using Adaptive Fine-Tuned Convolutional Neural Network." *IEEE Access*, 9, 41344–41359, doi:10.1109/ACCESS.2021.3065273

[19] Sil Kar, Sudeshna & Maity, Santi. (2017). "Automatic Detection of Retinal Lesions for Screening of Diabetic Retinopathy." *IEEE Transactions on Biomedical Engineering*, 65(3), 608–618, doi:10.1109/TBME.2017.2707578

[20] Qummar, S., Khan, F.G., Shah, S., Khan, A., Shamshirband, S., Rehman, Z.U., Khan, I.A., & Jadoon, W. (2019). "A Deep Learning Ensemble Approach for Diabetic Retinopathy Detection." *IEEE Access*, 7, 150530–150539. https://api.semanticscholar.org/CorpusID:204939227

[21] Pan, A., Yang, J., & Shi, C. (2024). "Research on Deep Learning-based Detection of Changes in Diabetic Retinopathy Lesions." In *Proceedings of the 2023 7th International Conference on Electronic Information Technology and Computer Engineering (EITCE '23)*. Association for Computing Machinery, New York, 1702–1707, https://doi.org/10.1145/3650400.3650684

[22] Ten Dam, W., Grol, M., Zeegers, Z., Dehghani, A., & Aldewereld, H. (2023). "Representative Data Generation of Diabetic Retinopathy Synthetic Retinal Images." In *Proceedings of the 2023 Conference on Human Centered Artificial Intelligence: Education and Practice (HCAIep '23)*. Association for Computing Machinery, New York, 9–15, https://doi.org/10.1145/3633083.3633175

[23] Lee, C.-H. & Ke, Y.-H. (2021). "Fundus Images Classification for Diabetic Retinopathy using Deep Learning." In *Proceedings of the 13th International Conference on Computer Modeling and Simulation (ICCMS '21)*. Association for Computing Machinery, New York, 264–270, https://doi.org/10.1145/3474963.3475849

[24] Shorfuzzaman, M., Hossain, M.S., & El Saddik, A. (2021). "An Explainable Deep Learning Ensemble Model for Robust Diagnosis of Diabetic Retinopathy Grading." *ACM Transactions on Multimedia Computing Communications and Applications*, 17(3), 1–24, https://doi.org/10.1145/3469841

[25] Beede, E., Baylor, E., Hersch, F., Iurchenko, A., Wilcox, L., Ruamviboonsuk, P., & Vardoulakis, L.M. (2020). "A Human-Centered Evaluation of a Deep Learning System Deployed in Clinics for the Detection of Diabetic Retinopathy." In *Proceedings of the 2020 CHI Conference on Human Factors in Computing Systems (CHI '20)*. Association for Computing Machinery, New York, 1–12, https://doi.org/10.1145/3313831.3376718

[26] Hatua, Amartya, Subudhi, Badri, Thangaraj, Veerakumar, & Ghosh, Ashish. (2021). "Early Detection of Diabetic Retinopathy from Big Data in Hadoop Framework." *Displays*, 70, 102061, 10.1016/j.displa.2021.102061

[27] Shakibania, Hossein, Raoufi, Sina, Pourafkham, Behnam, Khotanlou, Hassan, & Mansoorizadeh, Muharram. (2024). "Dual Branch Deep Learning Network for Detection and Stage Grading of Diabetic Retinopathy." *Biomedical Signal Processing and Control*, 93, 106168, https://doi.org/10.48550/arXiv.2308.09945

[28] Modi, Praveen & Kumar, Yugal. (2023). "Smart Detection and Diagnosis of Diabetic Retinopathy Using Bat Based Feature Selection Algorithm and Deep Forest Technique." *Computers & Industrial Engineering*, 182, 109364, 10.1016/j.cie.2023.109364

[29] Tabtaba, AhlamAsadig & Ata, Oguz. (2024). "Diabetic Retinopathy Detection Using Developed Hybrid Cascaded Multi-Scale DCNN with Hybrid Heuristic Strategy." *Biomedical Signal Processing and Control*, 89, 105718, 10.1016/j.bspc.2023.105718

[30] Yang, Jing, Qin, Haoshen, Por, Lip Yee, Shaikh, Zaffar Ahmed, Alfarraj, Osama, Tolba, Amr, Elghatwary, Magdy, & Thwin, Myo. (2024). "Optimizing Diabetic Retinopathy Detection with Inception-V4 and Dynamic Version of Snow Leopard Optimization Algorithm." *Biomedical Signal Processing and Control*, 96(Part A), 106501, https://doi.org/10.1016/j.bspc.2024.106501

[31] Pour, Asra, Seyedarabi, Hadi, Jahromi, Seyed, Javadzadeh, Alireza. (2020). Automatic Detection and Monitoring of Diabetic Retinopathy Using Efficient Convolutional Neural Networks and Contrast Limited Adaptive Histogram Equalization. *IEEE Access*, 8, 136668–136673, doi:10.1109/ACCESS.2020.3005044

[32] Ghouali, S., Onyema, E.M., Guellil, M.S., Wajid, M.A., Clare, O., Cherifi, W., & Feham, M. (2022). "Artificial Intelligence-Based Teleopthalmology Application for Diagnosis of Diabetics Retinopathy." *IEEE Open Journal of Engineering in Medicine and Biology* 3, 124–133, doi: 10.1109/OJEMB.2022.3192780

[33] Xiao, Z., Zhang, Y., Wu, J., & Zhang, X. (2021). "SE-MIDNet Based on Deep Learning for Diabetic Retinopathy Classification." In *Proceedings of the 2021 7th International Conference on Computing and Artificial Intelligence (ICCAI '21)*. Association for Computing Machinery, New York, 92–98, https://doi.org/10.1145/3467707.3467720

[34] Zhang, Zilin. (2020). "Deep-Learning-Based Early Detection of Diabetic Retinopathy on Fundus Photography Using EfficientNet." In *Proceedings of the 2020 the 4th International Conference on Innovation in Artificial Intelligence (ICIAI '20)*. Association for Computing Machinery, New York, 70–74, https://doi.org/10.1145/3390557.3394303

[35] Hossen, Md Sazzad, Reza, Alim Ahmed, & Mishu, Mahbub C. (2020). "An Automated Model using Deep Convolutional Neural Network for Retinal Image Classification to Detect Diabetic Retinopathy." In *Proceedings of the International Conference on Computing Advancements (ICCA 2020)*. Association for Computing Machinery, New York, 1–8, https://doi.org/10.1145/3377049.3377067

[36] Bansal, Vipin, Jain, Amit, & Walia, Navpreet Kaur. (2024). "Diabetic Retinopathy Detection through Generative AI Techniques: A Review." *Results in Optics*, 100700, https://doi.org/10.1016/j.rio.2024.100700

Chapter 8

Intelligent Applications for Medical Image Analysis

Srabanti Maji, Pooja Gupta, Pradeep Singh Rawat and Tripti Halder

8.1 Introduction

Medical imaging greatly benefits clinical applications, life science research, and other fields [1, 2]. Various medical imaging modalities map values to the airspace, create discrete images by sampling or reconstruction and convey an anatomical region's interior structure or function [3–5]. Every advancement in imaging technology, such as computed tomography (CT), magnetic resonance imaging (MRI), Positron Emission Computed Tomography (PET/CT), and x-rays, enhances and expands the observational capabilities of medical items [6–9]. It has been essential in raising medical standards and advancing medical capabilities [10]. The ability to analyse medical images has significantly increased with the advancement of computer science, and one of the key areas of machine learning (ML) research is deep learning [11]. The field of computer vision has witnessed impressive advancements in deep learning [12–14]. Deep learning applications for lesion target segmentation, localisation, detection, image registration, and fusion in medical images have also made significant strides. Quick diagnosis and significantly reduced diagnosis time [15].

DOI: 10.1201/9781003617013-8

Despite significant advancements in deep learning-based medical diagnostics [16–19], certain pressing issues remain in clinical practice.

1. The capacity of data-driven deep learning algorithms to generalise is frequently contested and questioned. The algorithm's performance will drastically decline in the event of insufficient sample data and discrepancies in training and real sample distribution. One of the aspects that has been questioned is whether the model trained in the situation of very few medical samples can be used for high-precision and sensitive medical image analysis, which is different from natural image processing with powerful datasets [20–23]. Due to subpar imaging technology in Indian hospitals, Google's deep learning algorithm for diagnosing diabetic retinopathy has encountered difficulties in Indian labs and hospitals, as the Wall Street Journal reported on January 26, 2019. The proposed algorithm cannot reliably identify low-quality photos.
2. Deep questions regarding how reliable deep learning is are brought up by adversarial examples. Instances that are marginally disrupted are known as adversarial instances, and they have a high probability of causing the model to produce inaccurate findings. The advent of this "ridiculous" phenomenon has compelled researchers to investigate deep learning techniques to produce reliable output.
3. Deep learning has an end-to-end prediction procedure and the ability to automatically extract abstract features. It is limited to direct results, without an aetiology, pathology, or diagnostic basis, and cannot be completely believed or accepted. In the case of glaucoma screening (refer to Figure 8.1), physicians can identify the disease by utilising intraocular pressure detection, visual field detection, and manual examination of the optic disc. These methods, when paired with the patient's clinical symptoms and pathological reports, enable them to determine the cause and pathology of the condition. However, due to a lack of process interpretability, deep learning uses neural networks to learn a large number of labelled sample data and extract features; as a result,

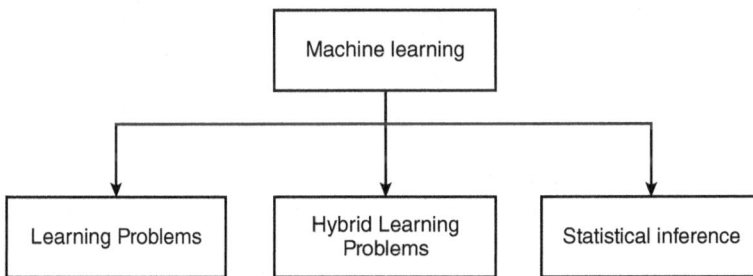

Figure 8.1   Various Categories of Learning.

the resulting model finds it difficult to support medical diagnosis or causal reasoning in medical research and struggles to explain the correlation or causal relationship between its input and output in clinical practice [24–28].

The development and application of deep learning in the field of medical image processing have made interpretability a challenging issue. Therefore, this article offers a thorough comparative review of cutting-edge artificial intelligence (AI) applications in medical imaging systems to overcome the aforementioned problems. These are

1. First, the application status, challenges encountered by deep learning in the medical field, and the trend of development of deep learning in medical image processing are evaluated.
2. The meaning of deep learning interpretability is explored, with an emphasis on the research techniques related to this concept.
3. Development and advancement in the field of deep learning interpretability, specifically in the context of medical image processing.
4. The research on deep learning interpretability in medical image processing is finally reviewed in terms of its development trend.

The rest of the article is structured as follows: Section 2 discusses the Background Work on Medical Image Analysis. The Role of Intelligent Systems in Medical Image Studies is covered in Section 3. The Deep learning architecture for medical image analysis is mentioned in Section 4. In Section 5, processes involved in medical image analysis are discussed. Trends and challenges in Medical Image analysis are provided in section 6. The paper is concluded along with future scope in Section 7.

8.2 Background Work on Medical Image Analysis

In a reasonably short amount of time, all deep learning applications, associated AI models, clinical data, and image investigation may have the greatest potential to positively and permanently impact human lives [1, 29]. Image retrieval, image creation, image analysis, and image-based visualisation are all involved in the computer processing and interpretation of medical images [2, 30]. Computer vision, pattern recognition, image mining, and ML have all become increasingly important aspects of medical image processing [3, 31]. One approach that is frequently utilised to provide the accuracy of the aft state is deep learning. Medical image analysis now has more opportunities as a result [4, 32]. A wide range of problems are addressed by deep learning applications in healthcare, including personalised therapy recommendations, infection monitoring, and cancer detection [5, 33]. Physicians have access to a vast amount of data nowadays from several data sources, including pathological imaging, genetic sequencing, and radiological imaging [6, 34]. Although we are all in a state of flux, the typical modalities used for medical imaging are PET, X-ray, CT, functional magnetic resonance imaging (fMRI), diffusion tensor imaging (DTI), and MRI to turn all this information into useful information [7, 8, 35, 36].

The various types of learning that an AI professional should be familiar with are listed below.

These are (A) Learning problems, (B) Hybrid learning problems, and (C) Statistical inference and Learning techniques.

1. **Learning Problems**: It can be performed by Supervised learning, Unsupervised learning, or Reinforcement learning

   a. ***Supervised learning***: Supervised learning represents a challenge in which a model is used to learn a representation between input samples and a target variable [26, 37]. Systems with examples of input vectors and the corresponding target vectors in the training data are referred to as supervised learning issues. When it comes to supervised learning, there are two main categories of issues: regression detection in classification and significant value identification in class marks [27, 38].

   b. ***Unsupervised Learning***: The employment of data relationship models to explain or eliminate data linkages presents certain challenges that unsupervised learning highlights. In contrast to supervised learning, unsupervised learning relies solely on input data and does not utilise target variables or outputs [33, 39]. Density estimation is said to as an unsupervised learning task that necessitates summarising the distribution of data. The cluster centres that can be located in the data are denoted by the letter k in the K-Means clustering algorithm [40]. Kernel Density Estimation is a type of density neural network that estimates the distribution of new points in the issue space using small sets of closely related data samples [34–38, 40–44].

   c. ***Reinforcement learning***: A person must master the use of feedback to function in a specific situation through a series of tasks known as reinforcement learning [45]. Even if feedback might be delayed, it is the same as supervised learning because the model can learn from some replies because it is systematically noisy, making it difficult for the entity and model to establish a causal relationship [46, 47]. Typical examples of reinforcement learning algorithms are temporal-difference learning, Q-learning, and deep reinforcement learning [48].

2. **Hybrid learning problems**: It can be performed by Semi-supervised learning, x, y

   a. ***Semi-supervised learning***: In the training data, there are many unlabelled cases and a small number of categorised instances; this is supervised learning [48]. Instead of using all labelled data as in supervised learning, the goal of a semi-supervised learning model is to make efficient use of all available data [49].

b. ***Self-supervised learning:*** To create a pretext learning assignment, such as anticipating context or rotating an image, the self-supervised learning system just needs unlabelled input [50, 51]. From there, an objective can be determined without supervision. Autoencoders, which are self-supervised learning algorithms, provide an excellent illustration. This kind of neural network is employed in the creation of a condensed or compact representation of an input sample [50–53].

c. ***Multi-instance learning:*** In multi-instance learning, individual examples in the collection are not marked; instead, the full set of examples is classified as either containing or not containing an example of a class [51, 53, 54].

3. **Statistical inference:** The process of coming to a conclusion or choosing a course of action is referred to as inference. Inference is used in ML to create models and make predictions [53, 54]. Various inference paradigms can be employed to elucidate the operation of specific ML algorithms or the resolution of related learning challenges. Inference is one method of learning, along with deductive, transductive, and inductive learning.

a. ***Inductive learning:*** Proof is used in inductive learning to evaluate the outcome. Using specific contexts, such as those that are general to all, to determine general results is known as inductive learning [55, 56]. Through a technique known as inductive reasoning, many algorithms are taught general rules (the model) by looking at specific historical precedents (the data)[55–58]. It's an induction strategy modified for a ML framework. The training dataset's tangible examples are generalised by the model. A model or hypothesis about the problem is developed using the training data, and it is assumed that the model will later apply to new, unknown data [57, 58].

b. ***Deductive inference:*** A deduction is the polar opposite of induction [54, 59]. In the same way that induction progresses from the person to the general, deduction progresses from the general to the specific [60, 61]. Induction is a bottom-up form of reasoning that uses the evidence available as proof for an outcome, while deduction is a top-down method of reasoning that seeks to fulfil all premises before determining the result [62, 63]. The algorithm can be used to make predictions before we use induction to suit a model on a training dataset, in the sense of ML [56, 58, 59, 61, 64–68]. The model is employed as a deductive method.

c. ***Transductive learning:*** The technique of anticipating particular examples from a domain is referred to in statistical learning theory as transduction, or transductive learning [63, 69]. It is not the same as induction, which is based on actual examples and entails learning universal laws [64, 70]. A new definition of inference is specified in terms of the model of estimating the value of a function at a particular point of interest. Observe that this principle of inference appears when one wishes to obtain the optimal result from a restricted amount of knowledge [71]. A well-known example is the k-near-est neighbours algorithm, which is used directly by the trans-ductive algorithm whenever a prediction is needed rather than modelling the training data [3, 47, 65, 71].

8.3 Role of Intelligent Systems in Medical Image Study

In the current scenario, there are various AI technique that provides key support in medical image study and analysis. The ML techniques include supervised, unsupervised, and reinforcement ML techniques. The study of medical images can be performed using three classes of techniques.

1. *Supervised Learning in medical image analysis*: Interpreting medical images correctly is crucial to making many disease diagnoses. Medical imaging is critically important to pathologists, radiologists, physicists, and researchers to diagnose patients and create novel treatment plans. However, because medical picture analysis done by hand is laborious and time-consuming, precise automated techniques must be found. Images are processed by ML algorithms in two steps. First, significant characteristics are extracted from the image using a manually developed feature extraction approach. In order to further classify the image based on feature extraction, a classifier method is used in the second stage. Consequently, it takes a lot of time and effort to analyse medical images using ML algorithms [66, 67].

    Medical picture categorisation, detection, and segmentation demonstrate remarkable performance from deep learning, particularly supervised deep learning, which has demonstrated capabilities that are on par with human performance. In medical image analysis tasks, deep learning algorithms have been demonstrated to outperform ML techniques [12, 67, 68]. Because deep learning algorithms can automatically extract features from images, they are more suited for automated medical image analysis and can yield precise diagnoses [68–70, 72]. Through the analysis of millions of photos, deep learning algorithms in image processing can be utilised to train models for automatic object identification. Both supervised and unsupervised learning apply to deep learning. In medical image processing, supervised learning has shown remarkable results, matching human performance [5, 68]. A ground truth dataset and previous information about the dataset's output are necessary for supervised learning. In order to effectively forecast the output, supervised learning aims to comprehend the relationships and structure of the input information. Medical image analysis uses both supervised and unsupervised ML techniques, each of which has advantages and disadvantages. The Feedforward Neural Network (FFNN), Recurrent Neural Network (RNN), Convolutional Neural Network

(CNN), Support Vector Machine (SVM), and others are popular supervised (deep) learning methods [71] (Jabeen et al., 2018).

2. ***Unsupervised in medical image analysis:*** Unlike supervised learning, unsupervised learning allows direct learning of a data pattern without the need for labels [15, 72]. The unsupervised learning understands and determines the inherent structure of a set of data points using statistical methods such as clustering algorithms and density estimation [15]. Unsupervised learning algorithms can be used not only for classification, detection, and segmentation but also for other tasks such as compression, dimensionality reduction, denoising, super-resolution, and reconstruction of images. A supervised learning algorithm cannot be employed directly in many situations when human supervision is insufficient, biased, or absent. The potential of the algorithms in supervised architecture is constrained in three ways: (i) Creating labels requires a significant amount of human labour; (ii) biases associated with the supervision process increase the likelihood that the algorithm will consider other worst-case scenarios when solving problems, and (iii) reduces the scalability of the target function.

In addition to grouping the data and extracting insights straight from it, unsupervised ML algorithms also employ these insights to make data-driven judgements. Furthermore, unsupervised models are more resilient since they serve as a foundation for a variety of intricate tasks, serving as the pinnacle of categorisation and learning. Actually, we execute a variety of tasks in addition to classification, including compression, dimensionality reduction, denoising, super-resolution, and some decision-making [71]. Unsupervised learning can be viewed as a preprocessing stage that prepares us for supervised learning tasks. In this case, unsupervised learning of a representation may improve classifier generalisation. The unlabelled data set is grouped in unsupervised learning according to underlying hidden features. We can learn something about raw data at least by using unsupervised learning to group the data.

One of the most well-known types of unsupervised learning is density estimation, which uses a different nonprobabilistic technique to uncover the inherent features and structure of big, complicated unlabelled data sets. Unlike parametric estimating, density estimation is a non-parametric technique with few limitations and distributional assumptions [73]. The usage of sensors and other imaging techniques in industry and medical diagnosis has increased dramatically. These techniques continuously record data and store it for subsequent analysis. When data are first recorded, there is a lot of redundancy or noise. Assume for a moment that an analyst sits down with all of this data to analyse it, leaving out all of the undesirable data and identifying all of the relevant variables and dimensions that contain the most critical information. This is a highly undesired dimension removal issue that requires dimension reduction treatment. The act of reducing a higher-dimension data set to a lesser dimension is known as dimension reduction, and it must ensure that the resultant reduced data succinctly conveys similar information. A few popular techniques for dimensionality reduction are as follows: Factor analysis and principal component analysis.

Unsupervised grouping of unlabelled data (patterns, data items, or feature vectors) into comparable groups is called clustering. Finding patterns in data through cluster analysis is explanatory in nature [74] (Jain, 2008). Semi-supervised clustering, ensemble clustering, simultaneous feature selection, and large-scale data clustering are a few clustering models that are evolving into hybrid clustering. It entails the study of multivariate data and is used in a number of scientific fields, including computer vision, ML, bioinformatics, picture analysis, and pattern recognition.

3. *Reinforcement learning in medical image analysis*: The image analysis process has been sped up and automated using numerous ML techniques. In contrast to the massive implementations of supervised and unsupervised learning models, there are still very few attempts to apply reinforcement learning to medical image analysis [75]. Even though reinforcement learning has been more popular recently, many medical analytic researchers still find it challenging to comprehend and apply in real-world clinical settings. Learning that uses reinforcement (RL) is neither supervised nor unsupervised. The largest expected cumulative reward is the aim of reinforcement learning [76]. Modern RL models have been used to tackle tasks such as video game playing, natural language processing, and autonomous driving that are challenging or impractical for conventional ML techniques. These RL techniques have shown exceptional results [77].

8.4 Deep Learning Architecture for Medical Image Analysis

The kind and quantity of issues that neural networks can answer have significantly expanded during the last 20 years thanks to the development of deep learning models [78]. Deep learning is a class of computations and regions rather than a single technique that can be used to address a broad range of problems. Although connectionist structures have existed for more than 70 years, contemporary designs and graphical processing units (GPUs) have elevated them to the forefront of AI. Neural networks' main architecture is depicted in Figure 8.2 [80].

In the deep learning architecture, the following layers make up a general deep learning architecture: combination layers, object detection layers, generative adversarial network (GAN) layers, output layers, normalisation, dropout, and cropping layers, convolution and fully connected layers, sequence layers, activation layers, pooling and unpooling layers, and normalisation layers [78]. The hidden layer (s) is the network's secret sauce. Their nodes/neurons allow them to model complicated

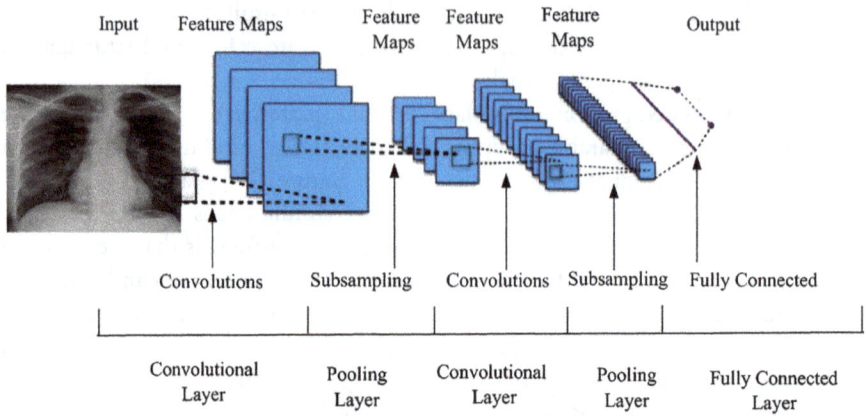

Figure 8.2 Neural network and deep learning's general architecture [79].

data. They are hidden since the training dataset does not know the true values of their nodes. Actually, all that is available to us are the input and output [80, 81]. Any neural network has at least one hidden layer. There is no legal requirement to multiply the number of inputs by N. There may be fewer hidden units in ideal circumstances than there are inputs [82, 83]. If you have a large number of training instances, we can employ several hidden units; however, when we have limited data, typically two hidden units will be sufficient.

1. ***Deep neural network (DNN):*** This architecture allows for nonlinear complexities in at least two layers. Here, regression and classification can be done. This model's remarkable precision makes it a commonly used advantage [84]. The disadvantage is that the error propagates back to the previous layer and gets low, making the training process difficult. Furthermore, the model learns too late [85].

2. ***Convolutional neural network (CNN):*** This model may work best with 2D data. This network comprises a fast-learning convolutional filter that converts 2D data into 3D with great performance. A large amount of labelled data is required for the classification procedure [86]. Nevertheless, CNN encounters problems such as human interference, sluggish convergence, and local minima. CNNs are being utilised more frequently to improve the effectiveness of human doctors in medical image processing since AlexNet's tremendous success [87].

3. ***Long short-term memory/gated recurrent unit networks (LSTM/GRU):*** Hoch Reiter and Schimdhuber created the gated recurrent unit network in 1997; nonetheless, it has recently gained popularity as an RNN engineering for many applications [88]. Instead of sticking with traditional neuron-based neural association models, the LSTM suggested the potential for a memory

cell [5]. As a portion of its data sources, the memory cell can store motivation for a brief or extended period, enabling the phone to evaluate its enormous value rather than just its most recent enlisted worth [89]. The gated recurrent unit was a 2014 development that enhanced the LSTM. The yield entrance found in the LSTM model is dropped in favour of two entryways in this model [90]. In some cases, the GRU performs similarly to the LSTM, but with less complexity, fewer loads, and faster execution [91].

8.5 Process Involved in Medical Image Analysis

Medical imaging plays a vital role in identifying, tracking, diagnosing, and assessing the effectiveness of therapy for many medical disorders. Artificial neural networks (ANNs) and deep learning are crucial for comprehending medical picture analysis in the field of computer vision. The Deep Learning Approach (DLA) is an emerging area of study that focuses on using advanced techniques to identify the presence or absence of diseases in many types of medical imaging, such as X-rays, CT scans, mammograms, and digital histopathology images. ML, a fundamental aspect of the AI revolution, presents new opportunities for the use of medical pictures in clinical practice. ML has shown comparable performance to that of medical professionals in identifying medical diseases based on medical imagery. ML has the potential to be crucial in achieving the goal of using AI in medicine, as software programs get certification for clinical usage. Nevertheless, despite the significant risks and thorough investigation into ML for medical pictures, it does not guarantee immediate advancements in clinical practice [92, 93].

The growing availability of biological information has required the creation of innovative methods, such as Translational Bioinformatics (TBI). This area combines the disciplines of biomedical data science and informatics to tackle issues ranging from fundamental biological research to therapeutic practices. The exponential expansion of high-throughput biologic data, including genomics, proteomics, and transcriptomics, has revolutionised the field by creating a wealth of data. Translational technology needs to adjust to this data, allowing medical practitioners to tailor choices for specific patients. ML approaches are used to process the information, discern significant attributes, decrease dimensionality, and detect patterns for ML-driven analysis. TBI and ML describe how they are used in different areas, examine their constraints, and evaluate medical image analysis techniques along a spectrum ranging from knowledge-based to data-based approaches. It emphasises the historical significance and present-day applicability of classical, knowledge-based AI methods and their compatibility with data-driven techniques such as deep learning [94, 95]. AI and bioinformatics play a vital role in healthcare, particularly in the field of precision medicine. AI is responsible for automating intelligent actions, whereas bioinformatics is the field that integrates biology, computer science, and statistics to analyse and understand biological data. These technologies can customise medical choices and treatments for both individual patients and whole populations. Image analysis is a basic opportunity to use digital pathology, enabling accurate and dependable data collecting. Photoacoustic Imaging (PAI) is a novel imaging technique that merges optical and ultrasonic imaging, providing excellent resolution, distinct contrast, and safety. Nevertheless, PAI encounters constraints in its practical implementation, including the compromise between depth and spatial resolution, as well as the need for enhanced imaging speed. Deep learning (DL), an innovative ML methodology, has been extensively used in the field of Precision Agriculture Imaging to enhance the quality of medical picture data. It explores the progress and uses of well-known deep neural network (DNN) architectures such as U-Net and GAN networks and examines the latest breakthroughs in the use of deep learning in PAI [96–98].

The medical industry is seeing a tremendous increase in the amount of data it deals with, which brings both new possibilities and difficulties in categorising and dividing unorganised sources of data. The integration of conventional statistical techniques with image processing technologies has been used to address medical issues. The expansion of data volume and image quality significantly influences advancements in AI, specifically in the field of deep learning methods for analysing medical data. Gaining insight into the transformation of ANNs into Deep Convolutional Neural Networks (DCNNs) is essential for comprehending large-scale data and making accurate predictions about future developments. It also seeks to elucidate the requirements of various phases in medical image processing by conducting a comprehensive review of existing literature. Additionally, it intends to give insights into studies that have brought about significant changes in the field and have successfully addressed medical issues connected to image processing utilising DCNNs. However, the heightened proficiency of medical doctors will allow for the analysis of new computer science problems from several perspectives [99].

8.6 Trends and Challenges in Medical Image Analysis

Medical image processing plays a significant role in radiology by enabling the identification of disorders from images. GPUs are used in diverse applications owing to their capacity to enhance parallel computing, their cost-effectiveness, and their energy efficiency. GPUs play a crucial role in medical imaging by facilitating the practical implementation of computationally intensive algorithms. It has fundamental operations such as filtering, interpolation, histogram estimation, and distance transformations. Additionally, it covers regularly used techniques including image registration, segmentation, and denoising. GPU implementations are tailored to particular modalities such as CT, PET, single photon emission computed tomography (SPECT), MRI, fMRI, DTI, ultrasound, optical imaging, and microscopy

[100]. In addition, it should be emphasised that computer-assisted diagnostic methods are capable of predicting the existence of both benign and malignant tumours via the analysis of CT images.

Furthermore, it has been shown that both traditional and deep learning-based systems possess the ability to perform a wide range of tasks, including preprocessing, liver and lesion segmentation, radiological feature extraction, and classification. Nevertheless, it emphasises the need for effective segmentation techniques that are compatible with a wide range of pictures. Additionally, it highlights the absence of research on unsupervised and semi-supervised deep-learning models for diagnosing liver illness. Subsequent investigations should prioritise the study of image fusion and the integration of crucial clinical and radiological characteristics to enhance the accuracy of categorisation [101]. Skull extraction from MRI scans is a vital field of study because of its significance in medical image analysis. Technological progress has resulted in the creation of diverse methodologies. The 3D U-Net design is used to partition the brain and separate lower-grade gliomas from stripped tissues, using a tiered technique. This technology has the capability to automatically remove and isolate gliomas from an MRI dataset of the human brain. When properly trained, this model surpasses previous techniques and may be valuable in predicting tumour stages because of its well-defined structure [102]. Three-dimensional medical image processing is a computationally demanding discipline that deals with a substantial volume of data. A pragmatic compute unified device architecture (CUDA) conversion procedure using Matrix Laboratory (MATLAB) code, while also comparing it to CUDA outcomes on three distinct general-purpose graphics processing units (GPGPUs). High-throughput GPGPUs are used to enhance the speed of several 3D medical image reconstruction techniques. Recent studies have concentrated on parallelising these algorithms by using new GPGPUs. The Katsevich CT image reconstruction technique also showcases the substantial improvement in medical image processing performance that can be achieved via the use of contemporary multicore and GPGPU processors.

Medical imaging is a very demanding application in terms of computing resources. Implementing an algorithm in parallel might be advantageous by using more processor cores and reducing memory use [103, 104]. Since its inception in 2014, the GAN has garnered considerable interest in the field of deep learning. The use of GANs has been shown to enhance the accuracy of medical picture segmentation by using its generative powers and data distribution capabilities. A comprehensive analysis of more than 120 architectures based on GANs for segmenting medical images was conducted before September 2021 and classified these research publications according to the areas of segmentation, imaging modalities, and classification techniques. This article examines the benefits, difficulties, and potential areas for further investigation regarding the use of GANs in the field of medical picture segmentation. The objective is to enhance the identification of medical professionals and patients by addressing issues such as instability, limited consistency, and lack of interpretability [105].

8.7 Conclusion and Future Scope

This chapter covers the basic introduction of the intelligent system's role in the process of medical image analysis. The process of medical image analysis follows the deep neural system for intelligent analysis. This chapter also covers the role of medical image analysis in the process of medical system improvement using AI approaches. The deep learning architecture plays a crucial role in taking the medical image input for decision-making and proactive measures for medical treatment. The medical expert can use the AI-based expert system for the detection and prediction of diseases. The images are preprocessed for further analysis and enhancement of the system. Hence the overall focus of the chapter covers the role of AI in the medical field and the study of the key processes and techniques used to solve the challenging concerns in the medical field.

References

[1] N. Chamoun, S. Matta, S. S. Aderian et al., "A prospective observational cohort of clinical outcomes in medical inpatients prescribed pharmacological thromboprophyl axis using different clinical risk assessment models (COMPT RAMs)," *Scientific Reports*, vol. 9, no. 1, Article ID 18366, 2019.

[2] T. M. Ali, A. Nawaz, A. Rehman et al., "A sequential machine learning-cum-attentions mechanism for effective sementation of brain tumor," *Frontiers in Oncology*, vol. 12, pp. 1–10, 2022.

[3] S. Abbas, Z. Jalil, A. R. Javed et al., "BCD-WERT: a novel approach for breast cancer detection using whale optimization based efficient features and extremely randomized tree algorithm," *Peer J Computer Science*, vol. 7, p. e390, 2021.

[4] M. Tsiakmaki, G. Kostopoulos, S. Kotsiantis, and O. Ragos, "Transfer learning from deep neural networks for predicting student performance," *Applied Sciences*, vol. 10, no. 6, pp. 2145–2218, 2020.

[5] L. Zhou, S. Pan, J. Wang, and A. V. Vasilakos, "Machine learning on big data: opportunities and challenges," *Neurocomputing*, vol. 237, pp. 350–361, 2017.

[6] M. Ghazal, M. Ghazal, A. Mahmoud et al., "Alzheimer rsquos disease diagnostics by a 3D deeply supervised adaptable convolutional network," *Frontiers in Bioscience*, vol. 23, no. 2, pp. 4606–5596, 2018.

[7] M. Upadhyay, J. Rawat, and S. Maji, "Skin cancer image classification using deep neural network models," in *Evolution in Computational Intelligence: Proceedings of the 9th International Conference on Frontiers in Intelligent Computing: Theory and Applications (FICTA 2021)* (pp. 451–460). Singapore: Springer Nature Singapore, April 2022.

[8] P. Hao, X. Zheng, and J. Z. Huang, "An effective approach for robust lung cancer cell detection," in *Proceedings of the International Workshop on Patch Based Techniques in Medical Imaging*, Munich, Germany, October 2015.

[9] R. Yan, F. Ren, Z. Wang et al., "Breast cancer histopathological image classification using a hybrid deep neural network," *Methods*, vol. 173, no. 3, pp. 52–60, 2020.

[10] J. Yao, Z. Lei, W. Yue et al., "DeepTy-Net: a multimodal deep learning method for predicting cervical lymph node metastasis in papillary thyroid cancer," *Advanced Intelligent Systems*, vol. 4, no. 10, pp. 2200100–2202235, 2022.

[11] S. Kanrar, and S. Maji, "A Study on Image Restoration and Analysis," in *Advance Concepts of Image Processing and Pattern Recognition: Effective Solution for Global Challenges* (pp. 35–61). Singapore: Springer Singapore, 2022.

[12] T. Chandrakumar, and R. Kathirvel, "Classifying diabetic retinopathy using deep learning architecture," *International Journal of Engineering Research and Technology*, vol. 5, no. 6, pp. 19–24, 2016.

[13] O. Biran and C. Cotton, "Explanation and justification in machine learning: a survey," in *Proceedings of the IJCAI-17 Workshop on Explainable AI (XAI)*, pp. 1–5, Melbourn, UK, January 2017.

[14] T. Miller, "Explanation in artificial intelligence: insights from the social sciences," *Artificial Intelligence*, vol. 267, pp. 1–38, 2019.

[15] X. Wang, Y. Chen, J. Yang, L. Wu, Z. Wu, and X. Xie, "A reinforcement learning framework for explainable recommendation," in *Proceedings of the 2018 IEEE International Conference on Data Mining (ICDM)*, pp. 587–596, Singapore, November 2018.

[16] G. Adomavicius and A. Tuzhilin, "Toward the next generation of recommender systems: a survey of the state-of-the-art and possible extensions," *IEEE Transactions on Knowledge and Data Engineering*, vol. 17, pp. 734–749, 2005.

[17] Y. Zhang and X. Chen, "Explainable recommendation: a survey and new perspectives," 2018, https://arxiv.org/abs/1804.11192

[18] R. L. Teach and E. H. Shortlife, "An analysis of physician attitudes regarding computer-based clinical consultation systems," *Computers and Biomedical Research*, vol. 14, no. 6, pp. 542–558, 1981.

[19] L. B. Smith and L. K. Slone, "A developmental approach to machine learning?" *Frontiers in Psychology*, vol. 8, p. 2124, 2017.

[20] Bińkowski Mikołaj, Danica J. Sutherland, Michael Arbel, and Arthur Gretton. "Demystifying mmd gans." *Proceedings of the International Conference on Learning Representations*, Vancouver, Canada, March *arXiv preprint arXiv:1801.01401*, 2018.

[21] Matthew D. Zeiler, and Rob Fergus. "Visualizing and understanding convolutional networks." In *Computer Vision–ECCV 2014: 13th European Conference, Zurich, Switzerland, September 6–12, 2014, Proceedings, Part I 13*, pp. 818–833. Springer International Publishing, 2014.

[22] Mahendran Aravindh, and Andrea Vedaldi. "Understanding deep image representations by inverting them." In *Proceedings of the IEEE Conference on Computer Vision and Pattern Recognition*, pp. 5188–5196. 2015.

[23] Liu Mengchen, Jiaxin Shi, Zhen Li, Chongxuan Li, Jun Zhu, and Shixia Liu. "Towards better analysis of deep convolutional neural networks." *IEEE transactions on visualization and computer graphics* 23, no. 1, 91–100, 2016.

[24] Ding Yongchang, Chang Liu, Haifeng Zhu, Jie Liu, and Qianjun Chen. "Visualizing deep networks using segmentation recognition and interpretation algorithm." *Information Sciences*, 609 (2022): 1381–1396.

[25] Olah Chris, Alexander Mordvintsev, and Ludwig Schubert. "Feature visualization." *Distill* 2, no. 11 (2017): e7.

[26] Bau David, Bolei Zhou, Aditya Khosla, Aude Oliva, and Antonio Torralba. "Network dissection: Quantifying interpretability of deep visual representations." In *Proceedings of the IEEE conference on computer vision and pattern recognition*, pp. 6541–6549. 2017.

[27] Fong Ruth, and Andrea Vedaldi. "Net2vec: Quantifying and explaining how concepts are encoded by filters in deep neural networks." In *Proceedings of the IEEE conference on computer vision and pattern recognition*, pp. 8730–8738. 2018.

[28] Kim Been, Martin Wattenberg, Justin Gilmer, Carrie Cai, James Wexler, and Fernanda Viegas. "Interpretability beyond feature attribution: Quantitative testing with concept activation vectors (tcav)." In *International conference on machine learning*, pp. 2668–2677. PMLR, 2018.

[29] Y. LeCun, Y. Bengio, G. Hinton (2015) Deep learning. *Nature* 521(7553):436–444. https://doi.org/10.1038/nature14539

[30] M. I. Razzak, Z. S. Naz, A. Zaib (2018) Deep learning for medical image processing: overview, challenges and the future. *Classification in BioApps: automation of decision making*. Springer, Cham, Switzerland, pp 323–350. https://doi.org/10.1007/978-3-319-65981-7_12

[31] S. Pang, X. Yang (2016) Deep Convolutional Extreme learning Machine and its application in Handwritten Digit Classification. *Hindawi Publ Corp Comput Intell Neurosci* 2016:3049632. https://doi.org/10.1155/2016/3049632

[32] F. Chollet et al (2015) Keras. https://github.com/fchollet

[33] Y. Zhang, S. Zhang et al (2016) Theano: A Python framework for fast computation of mathematical expressions, arXiv e-prints, abs/1605.02688. http://arxiv.org/abs/1605.02688

[34] A. Vedaldi, K. Lenc (2015) Matconvnet: convolutional neural net- works for matlab. In: *Proceedings of the 23rd ACM international conference on Multimedia. ACM*, pp. 689–692. https://doi.org/10.1145/2733373.2807412

[35] Guo Yanhui, and Amira S. Ashour. "Neutrosophic sets in dermoscopic medical image segmentation." In *Neutrosophic set in medical image analysis*, pp. 229–243. Academic Press, 2019. https://doi.org/10.1016/B978-0-12-818148-5.00011-4

[36] R. Merjulah, and J. Chandra. "Classification of myocardial ischemia in delayed contrast enhancement using machine learning." In *Intelligent data analysis for biomedical applications*, pp. 209–235. Academic Press, 2019. https://doi.org/10.1016/B978-0-12-815553-0.00011-2

[37] Rahmat Taufik, Azlan Ismail, and Sharifah Aliman. "Chest X-ray image classification using faster R-CNN." *Malaysian Journal of Computing (MJoC)* 4, no. 1 (2019): 225–236. https://doi.org/10.24191/mjoc.v4i1.6095

[38] Jain Govardhan, Deepti Mittal, Daksh Thakur, and Madhup K. Mittal. "A deep learning approach to detect Covid-19 coronavirus with X-Ray images." *Biocybernetics and biomedical engineering* 40, no. 4 (2020): 1391–1405. https://doi.org/10.1016/j.bbe.2020.08.008

[39] P. K. Sethy, S. K. Behera, P. K. Ratha (2020) Detection of coronavirus disease (COVID-19) based on deep features and support vector machine. *Int J Math Eng Manag Sci* 5(4):643–651. https://doi.org/10.33889/IJMEMS.2020.5.4.052

[40] A. K. Jaiswal, P. Tiwari, S. Kumar, D. Gupta, A. Khanna, J. J. Rodrigues (2019) Identifying pneumonia in chest X-rays: a deep learn- ing approach. *Measurement* 145(2):511–518. https://doi.org/10.1016/j.measurement.2019.05.076

[41] J. Civit-Masot, F. Luna-Perejon, M. Dominguez Morales, A. Civit (2020) Deep learning system for COVID-19 diagnosis aid using X-ray pulmonary images. *Appl Sci* 10(13):4640. https://doi.org/10.3390/app10134640

[42] N. S. Punn, S. K. Sonbhadra, S. Agarwal (2020) COVID-19 epi- demic analysis using machine learning and deep learning algo- rithms. https://doi.org/10.1101/2020.04.08.20057679

[43] G. E. Dahl, D. Yu, L. Deng, A. Acero (2012) Context-dependent pre-trained deep neural networks for large-vocabulary speech recognition. *IEEE Trans Audio Speech Lang Process* 20(1):30–42. https://doi.org/10.1109/TASL.2011.2134090

[44] Upadhyay Mayank, Jyoti Rawat, and Srabanti Maji. "Skin cancer image classification using deep neural network models." In *Evolution in Computational Intelligence: Proceedings of the 9th International Conference on Frontiers in Intelligent Computing: Theory and Applications (FICTA 2021)*, pp. 451–460. Singapore: Springer Nature Singapore, 2022.

[45] Y. Anavi, I. Kogan, E. Gelbart, O. Geva, H. Greenspan (2015) A comparative study for chest radiograph image retrieval using binary texture and deep learning classification. In: *Proceedings of the IEEE engineering in Medicine and Biology Society*, pp 2940–2943. https://doi.org/10.1109/EMBC.2015.7319008

[46] S. U. Akram, J. Kannala, L. Eklund, J. Heikkila (2016) Cell segmentation proposal network for microscopy image analysis. In: Proceedings of the *Deep Learning in Medical Image Analysis (DLMIA). Lecture Notes in Computer Science*, 10 0 08, pp 21–29. https://doi.org/10.1007/978-3-319-46976-8_3

[47] Maji Srabanti, Ajay Narayan Shukla, Vishakha Arya, and Pooja Gupta. "Object Detection Its Progress and Principles." In *2023 12th International Conference on System Modeling & Advancement in Research Trends (SMART)*, pp. 225–233. IEEE, 2023. 10.1109/SMART59791.2023.10428260

[48] S. Andermatt, S. Pezold, P. Cattin (2016) Multi-dimensional gated recurrent units for the segmentation of biomedical 3D-data. In: Proceedings of the deep learning in medical image analysis (DLMIA). *Lecture Notes in Computer Science*, 10 0 08, pp 142–151.

[49] M. Anthimopoulos, S. Christodoulidis, L. Ebner, A. Christe, S. Mougiakakou (2016) Lung pattern classification for inter- stitial lung diseases using a deep convolutional neural network. *IEEE Trans Med Imaging* 35(5):1207–1216. https://doi.org/10.1109/TMI.2016.2535865

[50] J. Arevalo, F. A. Gonzalez, R. Pollan, J. L. Oliveira, M. A. G. Lopez (2016) Representation learning for mammography mass lesion classification with convolutional neural networks. *Comput Methods Programs Biomed* 127:248–257. https://doi.org/10.1016/j.cmpb.2015.12.014

[51] J. Arevalo, F. A. Gonzalez, R. Pollan, J. L. Oliveira, M. A. G. Lopez (2016) Representation learning for mammography mass lesion classification with convolutional neural networks. *Comput Methods Programs Biomed* 127:248–257. https://doi.org/10.1016/j.cmpb.2015.12.014

[52] C. F. Baumgartner, K. Kamnitsas, J. Matthew, S. Smith, B. Kainz, D. Rueckert (2016) Real-time standard scan plane detection and localisation in fetal ultrasound using fully convolutional neural networks. In: Proceedings of the medical image computing and computer-assisted intervention. *Lecture Notes in Computer Science*, 9901, pp 203–211. https://doi.org/10.1007/978-3-319-46723-8_24

[53] Kanrar Soumen, and Srabanti Maji. "A Study on Image Restoration and Analysis." In *Advance Concepts of Image Processing and Pattern Recognition: Effective Solution for Global Challenges*, pp. 35–61. Singapore: Springer Singapore, 2022.

[54] A. BenTaieb, J. Kawahara, G. Hamarneh (2016) Multi-loss convolutional networks for gland analysis in microscopy. In: *Proceedings of the IEEE international symposium on biomedical imaging*, pp 642–645. https://doi.org/10.1109/ISBI.2016.7493349

[55] A. Benou, R. Veksler, A. Friedman, T. R. Raviv (2016) Denoising of contrast enhanced MRI sequences by an ensemble of expert deep neural networks. In: Proceedings of the deep learning in medical image analysis (DLMIA). Lecture Notes in Computer Science, 10 0 08, pp 95–110. 10.1007/978-3-319-46976-8_11

[56] X. Cheng, L. Zhang, Y. Zheng (2015) Deep similarity learning for multimodal medical images. *Comput Methods Biomech Biomed Eng* pp 248–252. https://doi.org/10.1080/21681163.2015.1135299

[57] A. BenTaieb, G. Hamarneh (2016) Topology aware fully convolutional networks for histology gland segmentation. In: Proceedings of the medical image computing and computer-assisted intervention. *Lecture Notes in Computer Science*, 9901, pp 460–468. https://doi.org/10.1007/978-3-319-46723-8_53

[58] M. Cicero, A. Bilbily, E. Colak, T. Dowdell, B. Gray, K Perampaladas, Barfett J (2017) Training and validating a deep convolutional neural network for computer-aided detection and classification of abnormalities on frontal chest radiographs. *Invest Radiol* 52(5):281–287. https://doi.org/10.1097/RLI.0000000000000341

[59] M. G. Ertosun, D. L. Rubin Automated grading of Gliomas using deep learning in digital pathology images: a modular approach with ensemble of convolutional neural networks. In: AMIA annual symposium proceedings, pp 1899–1908.

[60] J. Bergstra, Y. Bengio (2012) Random search for hyper-parameter optimization. *J Mach Learn Res* 13(10):281–305

[61] Y. Guo, Y. Gao, D. Shen (2016) Deformable MR prostate segmen- tation via deep feature learning and sparse patch matching. *IEEE Trans Med Imaging* 35(4):1077–1089. https://doi.org/10.1109/TMI.2015.2508280

[62] A. Birenbaum, H. Greenspan (2016) Longitudinal multiple sclerosis lesion segmentation using multi-view convolutional neural networks. In: Proceedings of the deep learning in medical image analysis (DLMIA). Lecture Notes in Computer Science, 10 0 08, pp 58–67. https://doi.org/10.1007/978-3-319-46976-8_7

[63] X. H. Han, J. Lei, Y. W. Chen (2016) HEp-2 cell classification using K-support spatial pooling in deep CNNs. In: Proceedings of the deep learning in medical image analysis (DLMIA). Lecture Notes in Computer Science, 10 0 08, pp 3–11. https://doi.org/10.1007/978-3-319-46976-8_1

[64] M. Havaei, A. Davy, D. Warde Farley, A. Biard, A. Courville, Y. Bengio, C. Pal, P. M. Jodoin, H. Larochelle (2016) Brain tumor segmentation with deep neural networks. *Med Image Anal* 35:18–31. https://doi.org/10.1016/j.media.2016.05.004

[65] M. Havaei, N. Guizard, N. Chapados, Y. Bengio (2016) HeMIS: hetero-modal image segmentation. In: Proceedings of the medical image computing and computer-assisted intervention. *Lecture Notes in Computer Science*, 9901, pp 469–477. https://doi.org/10.1007/978-3-319-46723-8_54

[66] S. Lu, Z. Lu, Y.-D. Zhang. Pathological brain detection based on alexnet and transfer learning. *J Comput Sci*. 2019;30:41–47

[67] R. Sa, W. Owens, R. Wiegand, M. Studin, D. Capoferri, K. Barooha, A. Greaux, R. Rattray, A. Hutton, J. Cintineo et al (2017) Intervertebral disc detection in x-ray images using faster r-cnn. In: *2017 39th annual International Conference of the IEEE engineering in medicine and biology society (EMBC)*, pp. 564–567. IEEE

[68] Q. Li, W. Cai, X. Wang, Y. Zhou, D. D. Feng, M. Chen (2014) Medical image classifcation with convolutional neural network. In: *2014 13th international conference on control automation robotics & vision (ICARCV)*, pp 844–848. IEEE

[69] L. D. Nguyen, D. Lin, Z. Lin, J. Cao (2018) Deep cnns for microscopic image classifcation by exploiting transfer learning and feature concatenation. In: *2018 IEEE international symposium on circuits and systems (ISCAS)*, pp. 1–5. IEEE

[70] J. Chang, J. Yu, T. Han, H.-J. Chang, E. Park: A method for classifying medical images using transfer learning: A pilot study on histopathology of breast cancer. In: *2017 IEEE 19th International Conference on e-Health Networking, Applications and Services (Healthcom)*, pp. 1–4. IEEE

[71] A. Jabeen, N. Ahmad, & K. Raza (2018). Machine learning-based state-of-the-art methods for the classification of RNA-seq data. *In Classification in BioApps* (pp. 133–172). Springer, Cham. https://doi.org/10.1007/978-3-319-65981-7_6

[72] A.O. Vuola, S. U. Akram, J. Kannala (2019) Mask-rcnn and u-net ensembled for nuclei segmentation. In: *2019 IEEE 16th international symposium on biomedical imaging (ISBI 2019)*, pp. 208–212. IEEE

[73] C.M. Bishop. (2006). Pattern Recognition and Machine Learning (*Information Science and Statistics*), 1st edn. Springer, New York.

[74] K. Jain (2010). Data clustering: 50 years beyond K-means. *Pattern Recogn. Lett.* 31, 8 (June 2010), 651–666. https://doi.org/10.1016/j.patrec.2009.09.011

[75] M. Hu, J. Zhang, L. Matkovic, T. Liu and X. Yang, 2023. Reinforcement learning in medical image analysis: Concepts, applications, challenges, and future directions. *Journal of Applied Clinical Medical Physics*, 24(2), p.e13898.

[76] Richard S. Sutton, and Andrew G. Barto. *Reinforcement learning: An introduction.* MIT Press, 2018.

[77] Ahmad E. L. Sallab, Mohammed Abdou, Etienne Perot, and Senthil Yogamani. "Deep reinforcement learning framework for autonomous driving." arXiv preprint arXiv:1704.02532 (2017).

[78] W. Sun, B. Seng, J. Zhang, W. Qian (2016) Enhancing deep convolutional neural network scheme for breast cancer diagnosis with unlabeled data. *Comput Med Imaging Gr* 57:4–9. https://doi.org/10.1016/j.compmedimag.2016.07.004

[79] S. Suganyadevi, V. Seethalakshmi, and K. Balasamy. "A review on deep learning in medical image analysis," *International Journal of Multimedia Information Retrieval*, vol. 11, no. 1, pp. 19–38, 2022.

[80] W. Sun, B. Zheng, W. Qian (2016) Computer aided lung cancer diagnosis with deep learning algorithms. *Proceedings of the SPIE Medical Imaging*, 9785, 97850Z. https://doi.org/10.1117/12.2216307

[81] Z. Xu, J. Huang (2016) Detecting Cells in one second. In: Proceedings of the medical image computing and computer-assisted intervention. *Lecture Notes in Computer Science*, 9901, pp 676–684. https://doi.org/10.1007/978-3-319-46723-8_78

[82] D. Yang, S. Zhang, Z. Yan, C. Tan, K. Li, D. Metaxas (2015) Automated anatomical landmark detection on distal femur surface using convolutional neural network. In: *Proceedings of the IEEE International Symposium on Biomedical Imaging*, pp 17–21. https://doi.org/10.1109/isbi.2015.7163806

[83] H. Yang, J. Sun, H. Li, L. Wang, Z. Xu (2016) Deep fusion net for multi-atlas segmentation: Application to cardiac MR images. In: Proceedings of the medical image computing and computer assisted intervention. *Lecture Notes in Computer Science*, 9901, pp 521–528. https://doi.org/10.1007/978-3-319-46723-8_60

[84] P.V. Tran, "A fully convolutional neural network for cardiac segmentation in short axis MRI," arxiv: 1604.00494, 2016, abs/1604.00494.

[85] Y. Xie, F. Xing, X. Kong, H. Su, and L. Yang, "Beyond classification: structured regression for robust cell detection using convolutional neural network," In: *Proceedings of the Medical Image Computing and Computer-Assisted Intervention. Lecture Notes in Computer Science*, vol. 9351, pp. 358–365, 2015, https://doi.org/ 10.1007/978-3-319-24574-4_43

[86] Y. Xie, Z. Zhang, M. Sapkota, and, L. Yang, "Spatial clockwork recurrent neural network for muscle perimysium segmentation," In: *Proceedings of the International Conference on Medical Image Computing and Computer-Assisted Intervention. Lecture Notes in Computer Science*, vol. 9901, Springer, pp. 185–193, 2016, https://doi. org/10.1007/978-3-319-46723-8_22

[87] T. Xu, H. Zhang, X. Huang, S. Zhang, and D.N. Metaxas, "Multimodal deep learning for cervical dysplasia diagnosis," In: *Proceedings of the Medical Image Computing and Computer-Assisted Intervention. Lecture Notes in Computer Science*, vol. 9901, pp 115–123, 2016, https://doi.org/10.1007/978-3-319-46723-8_14

[88] Y. Zhang, S. Zhang et al, "Theano: A Python framework for fast computation of mathematical expressions, arXiv e-prints," abs/1605.02688, 2016, http://arxiv.org/ abs/1605.02688

[89] Y. Guo, and A. Ashour, "Neutrosophic sets in dermoscopic medical image segmentation," *Neutroscophic Set Med Image Anal*, vol. 11, no. 4, pp. 229–243, 2019, https:// doi.org/10.1016/B978-0-12-818148-5.00011-4

[90] R. Merjulah, and J. Chandra, "Classification of myocardial ischemia in delayed contrast enhancement using machine learning," *Intell Data Anal Biomed Appl*, pp. 209–235, 2019, https://doi.org/10.1016/B978-0-12-815553-0.00011-2

[91] F. P. M. Oliveira, and J. M. R. S. Tavares, "Medical image registration: A review," *Comput Methods Biomech Biomed Eng*, pp. 73–93, 2014, https://doi.org/10.1080/ 10255842.2012.670855

[92] G. Varoquaux, and V. Cheplygina, "Machine learning for medical imaging: methodological failures and recommendations for the future," n.d., https://doi.org/10.1038/ s41746-022-00592-y

[93] M. Puttagunta, and S. Ravi, "Medical image analysis based on deep learning approach," n.d., https://doi.org/10.1007/s11042-021-10707-4

[94] P. Savadjiev, C. Reinhold, D. Martin, & R. Forghani, "Knowledge based versus data based: A historical perspective on a continuum of methodologies for medical image analysis," *Neuroimaging Clin. N. Am.*, vol. 30, pp. 401–415, 2020, https://doi. org/10.1016/J.NIC.2020.06.002

[95] N. Ahmad, P. Mohanty, N. Kumar, and E. Gandotra, "Machine learning in translational bioinformatics," *Transl. Bioinforma. Healthc. Med.*, vol. 13, pp. 183–192, 2021, https://doi.org/10.1016/B978-0-323-89824-9.00015-X

[96] N. Wang, and Q. He, "Artificial intelligence and bioinformatics applications in precision medicine and future implications," *Compr. Precis. Med. First Ed.*, vol. 1–2, no. 1–2, pp. 9–24, 2024, https://doi.org/10.1016/B978-0-12-824010-6.00058-7

[97] M. C. Lloyd, J. P. Monaco, and M. M. Bui, "Image analysis in surgical pathology," *Surg. Pathol. Clin.*, vol. 9, pp. 329–337, 2016, https://doi.org/10.1016/J. PATH.2016.02.001

[98] X. Wei, T. Feng, Q. Huang, Q. Chen, C. Zuo, and H. Ma, "Deep learning-powered biomedical photoacoustic imaging," *Neurocomputing.*, vol. 573, pp. 127207, 2024, https://doi.org/10.1016/J.NEUCOM.2023.127207

[99] S. Abut, H. Okut, and K.J. Kallail, "Paradigm shift from Artificial Neural Networks (ANNs) to deep Convolutional Neural Networks (DCNNs) in the field of medical image processing," *Expert Syst. Appl.*, vol. 244, pp. 122983, 2024, https://doi.org/10.1016/J.ESWA.2023.122983

[100] A. Eklund, P. Dufort, D. Forsberg, and S. M. LaConte, "Medical image processing on the GPU – Past, present and future," *Med. Image Anal.*, vol. 17, pp. 1073–1094, 2013, https://doi.org/10.1016/J.MEDIA.2013.05.008

[101] P. V. Nayantara, S. Kamath, K. N. Manjunath, and K. V. Rajagopal, "Computer-aided diagnosis of liver lesions using CT images: A systematic review," *Comput. Biol. Med.*, vol. 127, pp. 104035, 2020, https://doi.org/10.1016/J.COMPBIOMED.2020.104035

[102] R. Gupta, I. Sharma, and V. Kumar, "Skull stripping and tumor detection using 3D U-Net," *Mach. Learn. Big Data, IoT Med. Informatics.*, 71–84, 2021, https://doi.org/10.1016/B978-0-12-821777-1.00014-8

[103] A. Benquassmi, E. Fontaine, and H. H. S. Lee, "Parallelization of Katsevich CT Image Reconstruction Algorithm on Generic Multi-Core Processors and GPGPU, *GPU Comput. Gems Emerald Ed.*, pp. 659–677, 2011, https://doi.org/10.1016/B978-0-12-384988-5.00041-3

[104] J. W. Suh, and Y. Kim, "CUDA Conversion Example: 3D Image Processing," *Accel. Matlab with GPUs.*, pp. 193–231, 2014, https://doi.org/10.1016/B978-0-12-408080-5.00008-0

[105] S. Xun, D. Li, H. Zhu, M. Chen, J. Wang, J. Li, M. Chen, B. Wu, H. Zhang, X. Chai, Z. Jiang, Y. Zhang, and P. Huang, "Generative adversarial networks in medical image segmentation: A review," *Comput. Biol. Med.*, vol. 140, pp. 105063, 2022, https://doi.org/10.1016/J.COMPBIOMED.2021.105063

Chapter 9

Machine Learning Integration with Biomedical Problems

Suchi Johari, Abhilasha Chauhan and Navdeep Bhatnagar

9.1 Introduction

Biomedical combines principles of biology and medicine with engineering and technology to understand, diagnose, treat, and prevent diseases. It comprises a broad category of activities, from basic research to clinical applications. Key aspects of the biomedical field include biomedical research, biomedical engineering, Clinical Medicine, Public Health, Regenerative Medicine, Biomedical Informatics, and Biotechnology. Overall, the biomedical field is essential for advancing human health and disease understanding, developing enhanced medical technologies, and improving healthcare practices and policies. Biomedical problems encompass a wide range of issues related to human health and disease. These problems often involve complex interactions between biological, chemical, physical, and environmental factors. Some key areas of biomedical problems include: Disease and Disorders, Drug Development and Resistance, Diagnostics and Imaging, Medical Devices and Technology, Regenerative Medicine, Public Health and Epidemiology, Health Disparities, Mental Health, Aging and Geriatrics, and Environmental Health. These problems require interdisciplinary approaches involving biology, medicine, engineering, chemistry, and public health to develop effective solutions and improve human health outcomes [1]. Machine learning (ML) addresses various biomedical problems significantly [2]. With the help of large datasets, ML algorithms can uncover patterns and insights that contribute to better diagnosis, treatment, and

 DOI: 10.1201/9781003617013-9

understanding of diseases. ML is making an impact in the biomedical field: Disease Diagnosis and Prognosis, Genomics and Personalized Medicine, Drug Discovery and Development, Clinical Decision Support, Epidemiology and Public Health, Medical Research and Bioinformatics, Wearable Devices and Remote Monitoring, Automated Diagnostics and Robotics, Behavioral and Mental Health, and Advancements in Treatment Techniques. By harnessing the power of ML, significant advancements can be achieved in the field of biomedical research and healthcare for diagnosing diseases, developing new treatments, and improving patient outcomes, giving an opportunity for effective and personalized healthcare solutions.

9.2 Biomedical problems

Biomedical problems encompass challenges that healthcare professionals aim to address through various scientific and technological advancements in research (Figure 9.1). Some key biomedical problems include:

1. **Disease and disorder**

   In the context of biomedical science, diseases and disorders are often the focus of research, diagnosis, treatment, and prevention efforts. The diseases can be due to a wide variety of factors, including genetic, infectious, environmental, and lifestyle influences. Here are some key categories of diseases and disorders studied and addressed in the biomedical field: Infectious Diseases, Chronic Diseases, Genetic and Rare Diseases, Neurological Disorders, Mental Health Disorders, Autoimmune and Inflammatory Disorders, Endocrine Disorders,

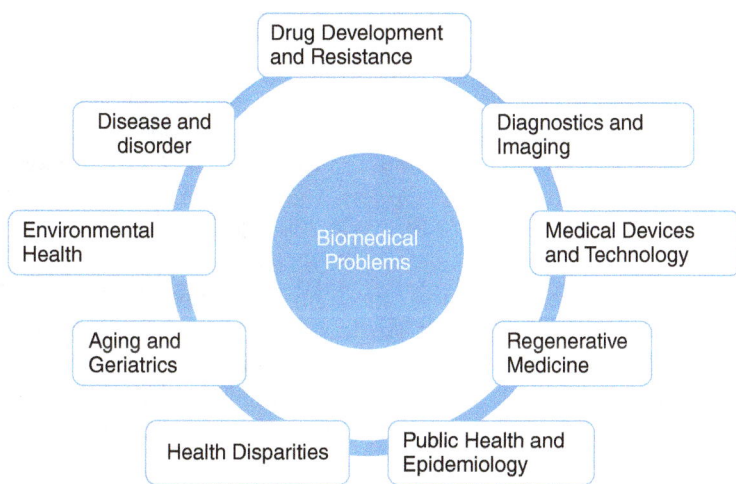

Figure 9.1   Biomedical problems.

Musculoskeletal Disorders, Cardiovascular and Hematologic Disorders, and Gastrointestinal Disorders. Biomedical research and clinical practice diagnosis mechanisms of these diseases and disorders, develop effective solutions and improve patient outcomes through prevention, early detection, and innovative therapies [3].

2. **Drug Development and Resistance**
Drug development and resistance are critical and intertwined aspects of biomedical science, particularly in the context of infectious diseases, cancer, and chronic conditions. Drug Development includes discovering drugs, testing and trials for clinical and preclinical, and approval of regulations. Drug Resistance involves Mechanisms of Resistance, Resistance in Infectious Diseases, Resistance in Cancer, Strategies to Combat Resistance, and Surveillance and Stewardship [4]. The interplay between drug development and resistance underscores the need for ongoing research, innovation, and vigilant monitoring to effectively manage and treat diseases.

3. **Diagnostics and Imaging**
Diagnostics and imaging are vital components in the diagnosis, management, and treatment of biomedical problems. They help in early detection, monitoring disease progression, and guiding therapeutic decisions. Diagnostics involves Molecular Diagnostics, Immunoassays, Point-of-Care Testing (POCT), Biochemical Tests, and Histopathology. Imaging involves x-ray, ultrasound, magnetic resonance imaging (MRI), polyethylene terephthalate (PET) scan, computed tomography (CT) scan, and mammography [5]. There are certain advanced imaging techniques that involve functional MRI (fMRI), SPECT, and Elastography. The integration of Diagnostics and Imaging in biomedical problems is crucial for accurate diagnosis, treatment, and monitoring of disease progression. Advances in these technologies continue to improve outcomes with precise and less invasive diagnostic options.

4. **Medical Devices and Technology**
Medical devices and technology help in diagnosing, treating, and managing biomedical problems. They range from simple instruments to complex machinery. Various medical devices and technologies are Diagnostic Devices, Therapeutic Devices, Surgical Devices, and Wearable and Portable Devices. Diagnostic Devices consist of Blood Glucose Meters, Digital Thermometers, Pulse Oximeters, Electrocardiogram (ECG) Machines, and Holter Monitors. Different Therapeutic Devices are Infusion Pumps, Dialysis Machines, Pacemakers, Defibrillators, and Ventilators. Surgical devices include Robotic Surgical Systems, Endoscopic Instruments, and Laser Surgery Devices [6]. The Wearable and Portable Devices are Wearable Fitness Trackers, Portable Electrocardiogram (EKG) Monitors, and Continuous Glucose Monitors (CGMs). There are certain advanced technologies such as 3D Printing,

Telemedicine, artificial intelligence (AI) and ML, and Nanotechnology. The integration of advanced medical devices and technology in healthcare has significantly improved patient outcomes, made treatments more effective, and expanded access to medical services. Continuous innovation in this field promises to further revolutionize healthcare, making it more precise, personalized, and accessible.

5. **Regenerative Medicine**
Regenerative medicine faces several challenges in the field of biomedicine [7]. These challenges are Immune Rejection, Ethical and Regulatory Issues, Limited Understanding of Stem Cell Biology, Tumorigenicity, Scalability and Manufacturing, Integration and Functionality, Aging and Senescence, Delivery Methods, Economic and Accessibility Issues, and Clinical Translation.

6. **Public Health and Epidemiology**
Public health and epidemiology play crucial roles in addressing biomedical issues. Biomedical challenges due to public health and epidemiology are as follows: a) Disease Prevention and Control that includes Vaccination Programs, Health Education, and Screening and Early Detection; b) Health Policy and Management that includes Policy Development, Resource Allocation, and Healthcare System Strengthening; c) Environmental Health that includes Monitoring Environmental Risks, and Water and Sanitation; and d) Global Health that includes Addressing Health Inequities, and Pandemic Preparedness and Response. Biomedical challenges due to Epidemiology are as follows: a) Disease Surveillance that includes Tracking Disease Incidence and Prevalence and Outbreak Investigation; b) Risk Factor Identification that includes Determinants of Health and Causal Relationships; c) Biostatistics that includes Data Analysis and Modeling and Prediction; and d) Intervention Evaluation that includes Clinical Trials and Public Health Interventions [8]. Biomedical challenges that are caused due to both public health and epidemiology are Chronic Diseases, Infectious Diseases, Health Disparities, Aging Population, Global Health Security, and Climate Change and Health. Public health and epidemiology are essential for understanding and addressing the complex biological, environmental, and social interactions that influence health outcomes.

7. **Health Disparities**
In the context of biomedical problems, health disparities manifest access to Healthcare, Quality of Care, Disease Prevalence and Outcomes, Social Health Determinants, Mental, Maternal and Child Health, and Genetic and Biomedical Research. Health disparities related to Accessing Healthcare are Geographical Barriers, Economic Barriers, and Cultural and Language Barriers [9]. Quality of Care caused health disparities include Provider Bias, Healthcare Infrastructure, and Patient-Provider Relationships. Disease

Prevalence and Outcomes include Chronic Diseases, Infectious Diseases, and Cancer. Social Determinants are Literacy, Employment and Working Conditions, and Housing and Environment. Mental Health disparities are Stigma and Discrimination. Maternal and Child Health-related health disparities include Maternal Mortality, Infant Mortality, and Childhood Health. Health disparities in Genetic and Biomedical Research cause underrepresentation in Research and Tailored Interventions. Efforts to reduce health disparities require a multifaceted approach such as Policy Interventions, Community Engagement, Education and Training, Research and Data Collection, and Improving Access.

8. **Aging and Geriatrics**

Aging and geriatrics present a range of biomedical challenges that require specialized approaches to address. The key issues in aging and geriatrics are as follows: a) Chronic Diseases and Multimorbidity that includes Prevalence of Chronic Diseases, and Multimorbidity; b) Cognitive Decline and Neurodegenerative Diseases that include Dementia, Alzheimer's Disease, and Other Neurodegenerative Disorders; c) Frailty and Physical Decline that includes Frailty Syndrome and Sarcopenia; d) Polypharmacy and Medication Management that includes Polypharmacy and Deprescribing; e) Mental Health Issues that include Depression, Anxiety, Social Isolation, and Loneliness; f) Sensory Impairments that includes Vision Loss, Hearing Loss, Management, and Adaptation; g) Bone Health and Osteoporosis that includes Osteoporosis, Prevention, and Treatment; h) Cardiovascular Health includes Heart Disease, Stroke Prevention, and Stroke Management; i) Geriatric Syndromes includes Falls and Incontinence; and j) Palliative and End-of-Life Care that includes Palliative Care and Advance Care Planning [10].

9. **Environmental Health**

Environmental health challenges are significant in the field of biomedicine, as they directly impact public health and the development of diseases [11]. Some key environmental health issues are as follows: a) Air Pollution that consists of Respiratory Diseases, Cardiovascular Diseases, and Neurodevelopmental and Cognitive Effects; b) Water Quality that consists of Contaminants and Access to Clean Water; c) Access to Clean Water that consists of Pesticides and Herbicides, Endocrine Disruptors, and Industrial Chemicals; d) Climate Change that consists of Extreme Weather Events, Vector-Borne Diseases, Food Security and Nutrition; e) Occupational Hazards that consist of Workplace Exposures, and Occupational Diseases; f) Soil and Land Pollution that consist of Heavy Metals, Toxic Waste, and Agricultural Contaminants; g) Radiation Exposure that consist of Ionizing Radiation and Nonionizing Radiation, and h) Noise Pollution that consists of Hearing Loss, Cardiovascular and Stress-Related Effects.

9.3 Advanced Technology in the Biomedical Engineering

Advanced technology in biomedical engineering has revolutionized healthcare. They are continually evolving, contributing to patient health, reducing healthcare costs, and advancements in understanding and treating diseases [12] (Figure 9.2). Some key advancements include:

1. **Medical Imaging:-** It provides detailed functional and anatomical information related to the human body [13]. Different types of Imaging Modalities Technologies are as follows: a) X-ray Imaging is used for diagnosing fractures, dental problems, and chest conditions; and b) CT-scan creates cross-sectional images of bones, vessels, and soft tissues. It provides 3D images used in diagnosing trauma, cancers, and vascular diseases; c) MRI creates detailed images of organs and tissues. MRI is useful for imaging the brain, spine, and musculoskeletal system, offering superior contrast resolution compared to CT; d) Ultrasound Imaging creates images of organs, tissues, and blood flow in real-time. It is noninvasive and widely used for imaging pregnancies, cardiac conditions, and abdominal organs; e) Nuclear Medicine Imaging involves injecting radioactive substances (radiotracers) into the body. It is used for functional imaging of organs and tissues, detecting diseases such as cancer, and evaluating organ function.

   a) **Advancements in Imaging Technology** is the introduction of High-Resolution Imaging, which has proved to be an improvement in detector technology and image processing algorithms have led to higher spatial resolution and improved image quality. Functional and Molecular

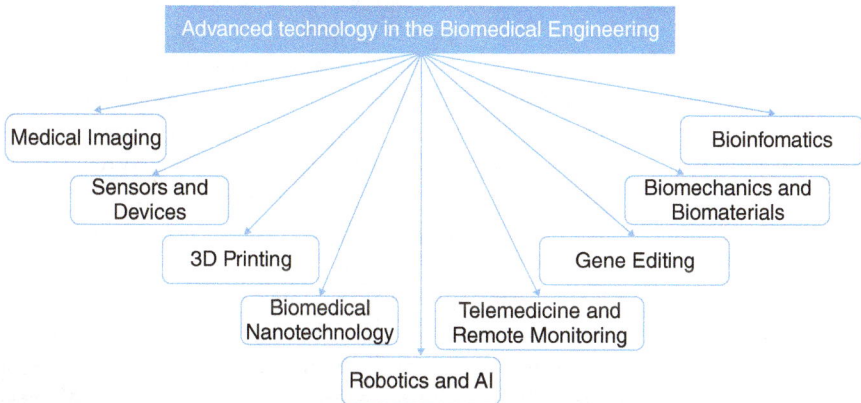

Figure 9.2   Advanced technology for biomedical engineering.

techniques such as fMRI, PET-CT, and single-photon emission computed tomography (SPECT) provide insights into organ function, metabolism, and molecular processes. Image-guided interventions provide integration of imaging with minimally invasive procedures allowing for precise targeting of treatments, reducing risks, and improving outcomes.

b) **Role of Imaging Technology in Biomedical Engineering** is Diagnosis and Disease Monitoring where medical imaging helps in the detection, characterization, and monitoring of cancer, cardiovascular, neurological, and musculoskeletal disorders and injuries. Imaging Technology also plays an important role in Research and Development for Biomedical engineers who use imaging technologies to develop and test new medical devices, therapies, and treatment strategies. Personalized Medicine can be prescribed using Imaging provides detailed patient-specific information for tailored treatment plans. Education and Training have a role in medical imaging as it is essential for training healthcare professionals and researchers in anatomy, pathology, and advanced imaging techniques.

Overall, medical imaging continues to evolve contributing to the diagnosis, treatment, and understanding of human health and diseases in biomedical engineering.

2. **Biomedical Sensors and Devices**: They are critical components in biomedical engineering, enabling monitoring, diagnosis, and treatment in healthcare. Different types of Biomedical Sensors and Devices are Vital Signs Monitoring used for measuring vital signs. Examples include wearable fitness trackers, blood pressure cuffs, and temperature probes. Glucose Monitoring devices for continuous or intermittent monitoring of blood glucose levels in diabetic patients. Cardiac Monitoring Devices for monitoring heart activity, including electrocardiogram (ECG or EKG) machines, Holter monitors, and implantable cardiac monitors. Neurological Monitoring Devices for monitoring brain activity and neurological conditions, such as electroencephalography (EEG) machines and neurostimulation devices [14]. Respiratory Monitoring Devices for monitoring respiratory function, such as spirometers for measuring lung function and pulse oximeters for measuring blood oxygen saturation. Implantable Devices includes pacemakers for regulating heart rhythms, implantable defibrillators for detecting and correcting irregular heartbeats, and neurostimulators for treating conditions such as Parkinson's disease. Prosthetics and Orthotics Devices that replace or assist in the function of missing or impaired body parts, such as prosthetic limbs and orthopedic braces.

a) **Technological Advancements in Biomedical Sensors and Devices are** miniaturizations that can be worn or implanted discreetly. Wireless Connectivity integration of sensors with wireless technology allows for real-time transmission and remote monitoring, enhancing patient comfort and healthcare efficiency. Biocompatibility materials science advancements of biocompatible materials reduce the risk of rejection or adverse reactions when devices are implanted in the body. Smart Sensors and AI Integration provide sensors equipped with AI, providing insights and alerts for healthcare providers and patients. Energy Efficiency provides the development of energy-efficient devices and power management systems extends battery life and reduces the need for frequent device maintenance or replacement.

b) **Applications of Biomedical Sensors and Devices in Biomedical Engineering** are Disease Monitoring and Management that is done through Biomedical Sensors. Remote Patient Monitoring monitors the patient's health remotely, reducing hospitalizations and enabling timely interventions. Clinical Research and Trials: Sensors collect data for clinical trials, evaluating treatment efficacy, and monitoring patient responses. Rehabilitation and Assistive Technology is achieved through devices like prosthetics and orthotics to assist in restoring mobility. Sports and Fitness are achieved through wearable sensors that are used to monitor athletes' performance, track physical activity, and prevent injuries.

Biomedical sensors and devices continue to evolve with advancements in technology, enhancing healthcare delivery. They are integral to biomedical engineering, contributing to innovation in diagnostics, therapy, and personalized medicine.

3. **3D Printing**: 3D printing is used for creating customized prosthetics, implants, and even tissues and organs. Types of 3D Printing Technologies are service level agreement (SLA) creates high-resolution models suitable for detailed anatomical structures and surgical planning. Sodium lauryl sulfate (SLS) produces strong and durable components for implants and prosthetics. Fused Deposition Modeling (FDM) extrudes thermoplastic materials through a heated nozzle, building up layers to create models and patient-specific implants. Bioprinting produces tissues and organs for drug testing and regenerative medicine [15].

a) **Applications of 3D printing in Biomedical Engineering** are Anatomical Models that facilitate surgical planning, education, and communication with patients. Surgical Guides that are customized guides aid surgeons in precise implant placement and complex procedures, reducing surgical time and improving accuracy. Patient-specific implants (e.g., cranial and orthopedic) and prosthetics (e.g., limbs and joints) can be tailored to match individual anatomy, improving fit and function. 3D printing is used in dental applications for fabricating dental crowns, bridges, aligners, and surgical guides in dentistry, enhancing efficiency and precision. Bioprinting is used for the creation of scaffolds and tissues with intricate architectures. In Drug Delivery Systems the 3D printing creates personalized drug delivery systems, such as controlled-release formulations and dosage forms tailored to patient needs.

b) **Advantage of 3D Printing in Biomedical Engineering** is Customization that enables patient-specific designs and solutions, improving treatment outcomes and patient comfort. Rapid Prototyping accelerates the development of medical devices and treatments, reducing time to market and costs. Integration with Imaging provides direct integration with medical imaging data, enabling precise replication of patient anatomy and pathology.

c) **Challenges and Future Directions of 3D printing** are biocompatible and meet regulatory standards for medical use. Quality Control establishing standards for quality assurance and validation of 3D printed medical devices and implants. Scaling and Accessibility addressing cost-effectiveness and scalability to make 3D printing technologies more accessible to healthcare facilities worldwide. Bioprinting Complexity advances bioprinting techniques to create viable tissues and organs with functionality for clinical applications.

3D printing has significantly impacted biomedical engineering by enabling innovation in patient-specific care, surgical planning, tissue engineering, and personalized medicine. Continued advancements in technology and materials are expected to further expand its applications and benefits in healthcare.

4. **Biomedical Nanotechnology**: Biomedical nanotechnology involves the application of nanoscale materials, devices, and techniques to address biomedical challenges. It enhances diagnostics, delivery of drugs, imaging, and therapeutic interventions. Nanoscale Materials are the combination of Nanoparticles, Nanofibers, and Nanocomposites [16]. Nanofibers and Nanocomposites are used in tissue engineering.

a) **Applications of Biomedical Nanotechnology in Biomedical Engineering**: This approach enhances therapeutic efficacy, reduces side effects, and improves patient compliance. Nanoparticles can act as contrast agents in MRI, CT, and fluorescence imaging. They improve imaging resolution and enable early detection of diseases. Nanotechnology enables targeted therapies where nanoparticles are functionalized to selectively bind to diseased cells or tissues. Nanotechnology incorporates nanomaterials that amplify signals or detect biomarkers with high precision. Nanotechnology develops biomaterials and scaffolds for tissue engineering. These materials provide mechanical support that promotes tissue regeneration and repair. Nanomaterials are used to coat or modify implant surfaces to improve biocompatibility, reduce inflammation, and prevent infections.

b) **Technological Advances in Biomedical Nanotechnology** are Surface Functionalization are technique that modify nanoparticle surfaces with ligands, antibodies, or peptides for specific targeting and interaction with biological molecules or cells. Multifunctional Nanocarriers for the development of nanoparticles capable of carrying multiple cargoes (e.g., drugs and imaging agents) simultaneously, allowing for theranostic applications. Nano-bio Interfaces optimize biocompatibility and minimize immune responses. Nanotechnology in Gene Editing offers potential treatments for genetic disorders.

c) **Challenges and Considerations in Biomedical Nanotechnology** are ensuring the safety of nanomaterials in biological systems. Addressing regulatory challenges and establishing standards for nanotechnology-based biomedical products. Scaling up production methods for nanotechnology-enabled biomedical devices and therapies.

Biomedical nanotechnology holds tremendous promise for advancing diagnostics, therapies, and regenerative medicine.

Robotics and AI: Robotics and AI have significantly transformed biomedical engineering by enhancing precision, efficiency, and capabilities in various healthcare applications [17].

d) **Robotics in Biomedical Engineering**: Robotic systems such as the da Vinci Surgical System are used for complex procedures through small incisions with enhanced dexterity and precision. Allows surgeons to perform surgeries remotely, expanding access to specialized care and expertise. Robots assist in physical therapy and rehabilitation, providing repetitive and controlled movements to aid in recovery from injuries or surgeries. Advanced robotic prosthetics replicate natural movements and provide sensory feedback, improving mobility and quality of life for amputees. Wearable robotic devices support and augment human strength and mobility, assisting patients with mobility impairments or enhancing performance in rehabilitation and industrial settings. Robotic systems automate processes in drug development, accelerating the identification of potential therapies. Robots handle samples, perform assays, and analyze data with high precision and reproducibility in research laboratories and clinical diagnostics.

e) **Artificial Intelligence (AI) in Biomedical Engineering**: AI algorithms predict, analyze, diagnose, and detect abnormalities. AI systems aid healthcare providers by offering second opinions and assisting in decision-making based on vast amounts of data. AI analyzes genetic data, biomarkers, and patient records for providing personalized treatment, prediction, and optimization. AI optimizes drug dosages and delivery methods based on patient requirements and treatment compliance, enhancing efficacy and reducing side effects. AI models predict patient outcomes, identify at-risk populations, and recommend interventions to improve healthcare delivery and patient outcomes. AI-powered Natural Language Processing (NLP) extracts information, supporting research and clinical decision-making. AI automates administrative tasks, scheduling, and resource allocation in healthcare facilities, improving efficiency and reducing costs. AI analyzes real-time patient data from wearables and medical devices to monitor health status, detect anomalies, and alert healthcare providers.

f) **Challenges and Considerations**: Data Security that ensures patient data confidentiality and protects against cyber threats. Ethical and Regulatory Issues address concerns related to AI decision-making, bias in algorithms, and accountability in healthcare practices. Integration and Adoption Overcomes barriers to integrating robotics and AI into existing healthcare systems, including cost, training, and acceptance by healthcare professionals and patients.

Robotics and AI are transforming biomedical engineering by advancing surgical capabilities, enhancing diagnostics, personalizing medicine, and improving healthcare delivery.

5. **Telemedicine and Remote Monitoring**: Utilizes communication technology for remote consultations, monitoring patients in real-time, and providing healthcare in remote or underserved areas. These technologies have revolutionized healthcare delivery, allowing for virtual consultations, remote patient monitoring, and the management of chronic conditions [18].

a) **Telemedicine**: The applications and impact of telemedicine in biomedical engineering are Virtual Consultations done through Remote Patient-Provider Interactions that enable healthcare providers to consult with patients remotely, facilitating access to healthcare services regardless of geographic location or physical mobility. Specialist Consultations allow specialists to remotely assist in diagnosing and treating patients in underserved or rural areas where specialized care may not be readily available. Telemedicine Technologies include Video Conferencing provided through Real-time audio-visual communication between healthcare providers and patients, enhancing communication and rapport. Remote Monitoring integrates medical devices and sensors to monitor vital signs, symptoms, and adherence to treatment plans remotely. Transmission of patient data to specialists for review and consultation at a later time.

■ **Applications of Telemedicine in Biomedical Engineering**: Telemedicine supports ongoing monitoring and management of chronic conditions through remote consultations and data tracking. Post-operative Care allows for follow-up visits and monitoring of surgical recovery remotely. Mental Health Services provides access to mental health professionals and counseling services remotely, addressing barriers to care and stigma associated with seeking help.

b) **Remote Monitoring**: The applications and impact of remote monitoring are Wearable Devices for Continuous Monitoring such as wearable fitness trackers, smartwatches, and medical-grade sensors that monitor vital signs in real time. Alert Systems to notify healthcare providers of significant changes in patient health metrics, enabling timely interventions and preventing complications. Technological Advancements include Data Integration through the platforms and systems that integrate data from multiple sources (e.g., wearables and electronic health records (EHRs)) for comprehensive patient monitoring and analysis. AI and Predictive Analytics to analyze remote monitoring data to predict health conditions, identify potential risks, and optimize treatment plans.

- **Benefits and Impact of Remote Monitoring** are improved access to care through telemedicine and remote monitoring bridge gaps in healthcare access, particularly in rural or underserved areas, and during emergencies or pandemics. Cost Savings reduce costs associated with frequent hospital visits, and travel, and provides early detection and intervention.

- **Challenges and Considerations of Remote Monitoring** are Regulatory and Legal Issues that are compliance with telemedicine regulations, licensure requirements, and reimbursement policies varies by region and can impact adoption and implementation. Technological Integration ensures the interoperability and security of telemedicine platforms and remote monitoring systems to protect patient data and maintain reliability.

Telemedicine and remote monitoring technologies are integral to biomedical engineering, offering enhanced healthcare, improving patient conditions, and promoting proactive health management. Continued advancements and integration with AI and wearable technologies hold promise for further transforming healthcare practices and addressing global healthcare challenges.

6. **Gene Editing**: Gene editing is a powerful technology in biomedical engineering that allows scientists to modify DNA within living organisms with precision. Different techniques of Gene Editing are clustered regularly interspaced short palindromic repeats (CRISPR)-Cas9 which utilizes guide RNA (gRNA) for DNA sequences, where the Cas9 induces DNA double-strand breaks (DSBs). This can lead to gene knockouts, insertions, or modifications [19]. It is versatile, relatively easy to use, and allows for precise editing of genes in a variety of organisms, including humans. Transcription activator-like effector nucleases (TALENs) designed proteins that can also be used for targeted genome editing. Zinc finger nucleases (ZFNs) engineered proteins bind specific DNA sequences and induce DSBs for gene editing.

- **Applications of Gene Editing in Biomedical Engineering** are Therapeutic Applications consisting of Gene editing holds promise for correcting genetic mutations responsible for inherited disorders. Gene editing can be used to modify cancer cells to enhance immune recognition or sensitize them to chemotherapy or other treatments. Editing genes to confer resistance to viral infections such as human immunodeficiency viruses (HIV) or hepatitis. Regenerative Medicine consists of Gene editing can modify stem cells to enhance their differentiation for tissue regeneration and repair. Organ Transplantation through Editing genes in animal organs to reduce rejection by the human immune system, potentially solving the shortage of donor organs. Research and Development can be done through Modeling

Diseases where Gene-edited animal models (e.g., mice) can mimic human diseases more accurately, facilitating research for potential treatments. Drug Development where Gene editing helps validate drug targets and test therapeutic interventions in preclinical studies.

- **Ethical and Regulatory Considerations** are Off-Target Effects where potential unintended mutations at sites other than the intended target, raising safety concerns. Germline Editing for editing genes in embryos or germ cells raises ethical dilemmas regarding safety, consent, and potential heritable changes. Equity and Access ensures equitable access to gene editing technologies and addresses concerns about genetic enhancement and inequality. Safety and Efficacy establishes guidelines and regulations for clinical trials and therapeutic applications of gene editing technologies. International Consensus addresses global governance and ethical standards for the responsible use of gene editing in biomedical research and healthcare.
- **Future Directions in the area of Gene Editing** are Precision and Efficiency achieved through the Continued advancements in gene editing technologies that aim to improve precision, specificity, and enhance safety. Therapeutic Innovations for further development of gene editing therapies to individual genetic profiles. Ethical and Societal Engagement for promoting dialogue and engagement with stakeholders to navigate ethical, social, and legal implications of gene editing technologies.

Gene editing has transformative potential in biomedical engineering, offering new avenues for treating genetic diseases, advancing Regenerative Medicine, and accelerating biomedical research. Balancing scientific progress with ethical considerations and regulatory oversight is crucial to harnessing the full benefits of gene editing while addressing societal concerns.

7. **Biomechanics and Biomaterials**: Biomechanics and biomaterials are foundational areas of biomedical engineering, focusing on understanding the mechanical principles of biological systems and developing materials that interact with living tissues [20].

a) **Biomechanics**: Biomechanics involves the study of the mechanics of biological systems, including tissues, organs, and the human body as a whole. It applies principles of physics and engineering to understand how forces and motions affect living organisms.

- **Applications of Biomechanics in Biomedical Engineering** are Orthopedic Biomechanics is a study of the mechanics of bones, joints, and muscles to design implants (e.g., artificial joints and bone plates) and orthotics (e.g., braces and prosthetics) that restore function and mobility. Cardiovascular Biomechanics analyze the blood flow dynamics, heart function, and arterial mechanics to develop devices (e.g., stents and heart valves) for treating cardiovascular diseases. Movement Analysis is the use of motion capture systems and biomechanical modeling to assess and improve movement patterns in rehabilitation and sports performance. Soft Tissue Mechanics is a study of the mechanical behavior of soft tissues (e.g., tendons, ligaments, and skin) to understand injury mechanisms and develop tissue-engineered constructs.

- **Techniques and Tools for biomechanics** are finite element analysis (FEA) which is a computational method for simulating the behavior of complex biological structures under various conditions, aiding in device design and surgical planning. Biomechanical Testing is an experimental technique (e.g., tensile testing and compression testing) to quantify the mechanical properties of biological structures. Motion Analysis technologies such as 3D motion capture systems and force platforms to analyze human movement for clinical and research purposes.

b) **Biomaterials**: They can be synthetic or natural in origin to perform specific functions when used in contact with biological tissues. Different types of biomaterials are metals used in orthopedic implants and dental applications due to their strength and biocompatibility. Biodegradable polymers (e.g., participatory learning and action (PLA) and patient global assessment (PGA)) are used for drug delivery systems, tissue scaffolds, and sutures. Ceramics such as hydroxyapatite are used in bone grafts and also for dental implants due to their similarity to natural bone minerals. Composite Materials are combinations of two or more materials to achieve desired mechanical and biological properties for specific applications.

- **Applications of Biomaterials in Biomedical Engineering** are Implants and Prosthetics that include Biomaterials used to fabricate implants (e.g., hip implants and dental implants) and prosthetics (e.g., limbs and joints) that integrate with biological tissues and improve patient outcomes. Tissue engineering for biomaterial scaffolds provides structural support for cells to grow and differentiate into functional tissues, advancing regenerative medicine approaches. Diagnostic Tools include biomaterial-based sensors and imaging agents for detecting biomarkers and monitoring physiological parameters in real-time.

- **Emerging Trends and Future Directions of biomaterials** are Personalized Medicine that are customization of biomaterials and implants. Bioactive and Smart Materials for the development of biomaterials that respond to biological cues or stimuli (e.g., pH and temperature) for controlled drug release and tissue regeneration. Bioprinting for integration of biomaterials with 3D printing technologies to create complex tissue constructs and organ models for research and clinical applications. Regulatory and Safety Considerations for ensuring biocompatibility, stability, and safety of biomaterials through rigorous testing and adherence to regulatory standards.

Biomechanics and biomaterials are integral to advancing biomedical engineering, enabling innovations in medical devices, tissue engineering, and personalized medicine. Continued research and interdisciplinary collaboration are essential to address healthcare challenges and improve patient care through innovative biomechanical solutions and biomaterial developments.

8. **Bioinformatics**: It integrates computational and statistical methods to analyze biological data, decipher biological processes, and accelerate discoveries in healthcare and medicine [21]. It develops algorithms, databases, and tools to extract meaningful insights from large datasets.

   ■ **Applications of Bioinformatics in Biomedical Engineering** are Genomics and Personalized Medicine where bioinformatics tools analyze genomic data. It studies gene expression patterns to understand disease mechanisms, identify biomarkers, and develop targeted therapies. Proteomics is the analysis of protein structures and functions to elucidate biological pathways, drug interactions, and disease mechanisms. Metabolomics is a study of small molecules (metabolites) in biological samples to identify metabolic pathways, biomarkers, and therapeutic targets. Clinical Informatics is an integration of clinical data with genomic and molecular data for precision medicine applications.

   ■ **Bioinformatics Tools and Techniques** include Sequence Alignment and Analysis, which are algorithms and software tools to identify similarities, mutations, and functional elements. Structural Bioinformatics for prediction of protein structures, interactions, and functions using computational modeling and simulation techniques. Application of data mining algorithms and ML models to analyze complex biological datasets, predict outcomes, and discover patterns. Network Analysis for visualization and analysis of biological networks to understand system-level behaviors.

   ■ **Significance of bioinformatics in Biomedical Engineering** is Drug Discovery and Development for Virtual Screening, which includes Computational methods to identify potential drug candidates by simulating interactions between molecules and biological targets. Pharmacogenomics for analysis of genetic variations to optimize drug efficacy and safety based on individual patient profiles. Disease Diagnosis and Biomarker Discovery includes Diagnostic Biomarkers for early detection, diagnosis, and monitoring of diseases (e.g., cancer and cardiovascular disorders). Predictive Models for the development of predictive models using clinical and molecular data to assess disease progression and treatment response. Precision Medicine includes Targeted Therapies for the use of genomic and molecular data to match patients with treatments tailored to their genetic profiles and disease characteristics. Clinical Decision Support for integration of bioinformatics tools in clinical settings to assist in treatment decisions and patient management.

- **Challenges and Future Directions in Bioinformatics** are Big Data Management for handling and analyzing large-scale biological datasets requires robust computational infrastructure and data management strategies. Interdisciplinary Collaboration for enhancing collaboration between bioinformaticians, biologists, clinicians, and engineers to translate bioinformatics discoveries into clinical applications. Ethical and Privacy Concerns for addressing issues of data privacy, consent, and genomic and personal health information.

Bioinformatics is pivotal in advancing biomedical engineering by providing computational tools and insights that drive innovation in genomics, personalized medicine, drug discovery, and clinical decision-making. Continued advancements in bioinformatics hold promise for improving healthcare outcomes and addressing global health challenges through data-driven approaches.

9.4 Machine Learning in Biomedical Engineering

ML has become increasingly important in biomedical engineering due to its potential to analyze huge data and extract meaningful insights that can improve healthcare outcomes [22]. Overall, ML has revolutionized biomedical engineering improving patient outcomes and advancing medical research.

Here are some key areas where ML is making an impact in biomedical engineering:

1. **ML for Medical Imaging and Diagnostics**: ML algorithms are used for the detection, segmentation, and classification of diseases. For example, ML models early detect tumors or abnormalities in medical images. ML has revolutionized the interpretation and utilization of medical images for diagnosis and treatment [23]. ML algorithms segment images to identify and delineate structures, such as tumors, organs, or blood vessels. This segmentation helps in precise localization and measurement, aiding in treatment planning and monitoring. ML models are trained to classify medical images based on patterns and features. For example, they can distinguish between different types of cancerous and noncancerous lesions, or between various stages of disease progression. ML techniques enable the detection of specific features within medical images, such as nodules in lung CT scans or micro-calcifications in mammograms. This assists radiologists in identifying potential abnormalities that may require further investigation. ML enhances the image quality through noise reduction, resolution enhancement, and image reconstruction from limited data. This capability is particularly valuable in scenarios where imaging conditions are suboptimal. ML is used for the quantitative analysis of medical images for the extraction of numerical data related to tissue characteristics, growth rates, or response to treatment. This objective analysis supports clinical decision-making and longitudinal monitoring of patients.

ML-powered diagnostic tools can provide automated preliminary assessments or second opinions based on image analysis. This can improve diagnostic accuracy, reduce interpretation time, and support radiologists in complex cases. ML models integrated with EHR systems can correlate imaging findings with clinical data, providing a holistic view of patient health history and aiding in comprehensive diagnosis and treatment planning. ML algorithms is used for the prediction of patient outcomes based on imaging data, such as prognosis after treatment or likelihood of disease recurrence. This predictive capability helps tailor personalized treatment strategies. ML techniques applied to imaging data support research initiatives by facilitating large-scale analysis, identifying imaging biomarkers, and uncovering new insights into disease mechanisms. ML in medical imaging faces challenges such as data variability, interpretability of results, and ensuring algorithm robustness across diverse patient populations. Addressing these challenges requires rigorous validation, ethical considerations, and continuous refinement of algorithms.

In conclusion, ML is transforming medical imaging and diagnostics by enhancing accuracy, efficiency, and the depth of information extracted from images. These advancements contribute to improved patient care, early disease detection, and personalized treatment strategies in healthcare.

2. **ML for Personalized Medicine**: ML techniques analyze genomic and proteomic data to tailor medical treatment and interventions according to individual patient characteristics. ML advances personalized medicine, which aims to improve medical treatment based on individual characteristics, thereby optimizing outcomes and minimizing adverse effects. Genomic data is analyzed by the ML algorithms to identify disease variations, response to a drug, and susceptibility. This enables clinicians to predict the risk of developing medical conditions and personalize treatment strategies based on genetic profiles. ML models integrate genetic and clinical data to predict an individual's risk of developing medical conditions. This prediction supports early intervention and preventive measures, improving overall health outcomes. ML algorithms predicts individuals respond to medications. This information guides clinicians in selecting the most effective drugs and optimal dosages for each patient, reducing adverse drug reactions and enhancing therapeutic efficacy. The patient data is analyzed by the ML-powered systems to provide personalized recommendations and assists in diagnosis, treatment planning, and monitoring of patient progress. ML techniques cluster patients into subgroups based on biomarkers, genetic profiles, or disease characteristics. This stratification improves the outcomes of clinical trials by identifying responsive patient populations and optimizing treatment efficacy evaluation. ML algorithms analyze data to monitor individual health metrics. This enables detection of health deviations, prompting timely interventions and personalized health management plans. ML facilitates the integration of diverse datasets,

including EHRs, imaging, genomic, and patient outcomes and data. By synthesizing this information, clinicians gain comprehensive insights into health status and can make personalized decisions. Implementing ML in personalized medicine requires address challenges of data privacy, ethical challenges related to data usage, regulatory compliance, and the need for robust validation of algorithms in diverse patient populations [24].

Overall, ML in personalized medicine holds promise for transforming healthcare by enabling precise, individualized treatment approaches that improve patient outcomes, enhance treatment efficacy, and support proactive health management. As technologies and methodologies evolves, ML plays an increasingly integral role in advancing personalized medicine practices.

3. **ML for Drug Discovery and Development**: They analyzes molecular structures, drug prediction, and optimization. This accelerates the process of discovering new drugs and reducing the cost of drug development. ML algorithms analyze data to identify drugs involved in disease cure. By prediction of target interactions and pathways, ML helps prioritize targets for further investigation. ML models screen large databases of molecules to identify compounds with potential therapeutic activity against specific targets [25]. Virtual screening methods, combined with molecular docking simulations, predict how molecules bind to target proteins, guiding the selection of lead compounds for experimental validation. ML models predict pharmacokinetic profiles and potential adverse effects early in the drug development process, optimizing candidate selection and reducing costly failures in later stages. ML-driven generative models, such as deep learning-based neural networks, generate novel molecular structures with desired properties. These models learn from existing chemical databases and optimize molecular properties (e.g., potency, selectivity, solubility) to design potential drug candidates. ML algorithms analyze existing drug databases, genomic data, and clinical outcomes. This approach improves drug timelines and reduces costs by leveraging existing safety and efficacy data. These predictive analytics optimize clinical trial design by identifying responsive patient populations, stratifying patients for personalized treatment approaches, and improving recruitment and retention strategies. ML-powered NLP tools extract and analyze information from vast biomedical literature and patent databases. This enables researchers to stay updated on current research trends, identify potential drug targets, and generate hypotheses for further exploration. ML in drug discovery faces challenges interpretability of models, and the integration of diverse data types. Ensuring regulatory compliance, ethical considerations, and validation of ML models in real-world scenarios are critical for successful implementation.

In conclusion, as ML techniques continue to advance, they hold promise for revolutionizing the pharmaceutical industry and improving global healthcare outcomes.

4. **ML for Healthcare Management**: ML models analyze EHRs to predict patient disease, optimize hospital operations, and improve diagnosis. This provides better resource allocation and patient care. ML is increasingly applied in healthcare management to optimize operations and enhance efficiency. ML models analyze data of the patient from electronic EHRs, including clinical history, lab results, and demographics, to predict patient outcomes such as readmission rates, complications, and response to treatments [26]. This information helps healthcare providers proactively manage patient care and allocate resources effectively. ML algorithms optimize the data of the hospital by predicting patient count, bed occupancy, and staffing requirements based on historical data and current patient conditions. This enables hospitals to streamline operations, reduce wait times, and improve patient access to care. ML techniques analyze activities in billing and insurance claims. This helps organizations mitigate financial losses and maintain compliance with regulatory standards. ML-powered systems automate routine administrative processes, such as appointment scheduling, processing medical records, and inventory management. ML models analyze population-level data to identify critical patient groups, disease outbreaks prediction, and preventive measure implementation. This approach enhances population health issues and reduces costs associated with chronic diseases. ML-based clinical decision support systems incorporate the knowledge of the medical field with the data of the patient and assist in diagnosis, planning of the treatment, management of medication, improved decision, and safety of the patient. ML algorithms analyze patient preferences, behaviors, and health data from wearable devices to personalize patient engagement strategies. This includes remote monitoring, personalized health coaching, and tailored treatment plans. ML techniques analyze healthcare quality metrics, patient feedback, and adverse event data to identify areas for improvement in clinical practices and patient safety protocols. This continuous feedback loop helps healthcare organizations enhance care delivery and mitigate risks. ML enables remote monitoring of patients through telemedicine platforms, analyzing real-time data to monitor vital signs, detect abnormalities, and intervene when necessary. This improves access to healthcare services in remote areas. Implementing ML in healthcare management requires addressing ethical concerns. Regulatory compliance ensures that ML applications meet legal and ethical standards for healthcare delivery.

In summary, ML is transforming healthcare management by leveraging data-driven insights to optimize operations, improve patient care quality, and drive efficiencies across the healthcare ecosystem. ML technologies hold promise for further enhancing healthcare delivery and patient outcomes globally.

5. **ML for Health Monitoring and Wearable Devices**: They analyze data from wearable devices for vital signs monitoring, anomaly detection, and real-time feedback to patients and healthcare providers. ML is playing a pivotal role

in health monitoring and wearable devices, transforming how individuals track their health metrics and enabling providers to deliver more care [27]. ML algorithms analyze real-time data from smartwatches, fitness trackers, and medical sensors. They monitor vital signs such as heart rate variability, blood pressure, glucose levels, and sleep patterns, providing individuals with actionable insights into their health status. ML models detect modifications in health metrics that indicate early signs of health problems or deviations from normal patterns. For example, ML algorithms can identify irregular heart rhythms (arrhythmias) based on ECG data collected by wearable devices, prompting timely medical intervention. ML-powered health monitoring systems personalize health recommendations based on individual health data and behavior patterns. This includes suggestions for physical activity levels, modifications of diet, reminders for medication, and management of stress tailored to each user. Wearable devices equipped with ML algorithms can detect falls or sudden movements indicative of emergencies, such as seizures or accidents. They can automatically alert emergency services, facilitating rapid response and improving safety for individuals, particularly the elderly or those with chronic conditions. ML enables continuous monitoring of diabetes, hypertension, and respiratory conditions. By analyzing trends in health data over time, ML algorithms provide insights into disease progression, medication effectiveness, and adherence to treatment plans. ML techniques analyze user behavior data, such as activity levels, sleep patterns, and dietary habits, to generate insights into lifestyle choices and their impact on health outcomes. This information helps individuals make informed decisions to improve their overall well-being. ML-powered wearable devices integrate with EHR systems to provide healthcare providers with comprehensive patient health data. This seamless data integration supports clinical decision-making, enables proactive healthcare interventions, and enhances continuity of care. ML approaches support postoperative care, chronic disease management, and personalized treatment adjustments based on real-time data. ML algorithms in wearable devices analyze fitness metrics, such as exercise intensity, calorie expenditure, and performance trends. They provide personalized workout recommendations and motivational feedback to users, encouraging physical activity and overall fitness. Implementing ML in health monitoring requires to protection of sensitive health information.

In conclusion, ML is revolutionizing health monitoring and wearable devices by enabling personalized, proactive healthcare management. By harnessing the power of ML algorithms, individuals can monitor their health in real-time, while healthcare providers gain valuable insights for delivering personalized care and improving health outcomes.

6. **ML for Robotics and Prosthetics**: ML techniques are used to develop intelligent prosthetic devices and robotic-assisted surgeries, enhancing mobility and surgical precision. ML is playing a transformative role in robotics and

prosthetics, enhancing mobility, autonomy, and functionality for individuals with disabilities and advancing the capabilities of robotic systems [28]. ML algorithms are used to interpret signals from electromyography (EMG) sensors, brain-computer interfaces (BCIs), or residual limb movements. This enables intuitive control of prosthetic limbs, allowing users to perform complex movements with greater precision and naturalness. ML models analyze gait patterns and biomechanical data to assess movement disorders, monitor rehabilitation progress, and customize prosthetic fittings. This personalized approach improves mobility outcomes for amputees and individuals undergoing rehabilitation. ML techniques integrate data from various sensors (such as cameras, light detection and ranging (LiDAR), and inertial measurement units) to enhance robotic perception and environmental awareness. This enables robots and prosthetic devices to navigate complex environments, avoid obstacles, and interact safely with humans. ML algorithms adaptively adjust assistive devices, such as exoskeletons and robotic orthoses, based on real-time user feedback and physiological measurements. This enhances comfort, reduces fatigue, and optimizes device performance to support daily activities and mobility. ML-driven design optimization techniques generate prosthetic designs that are customized to individual anatomical characteristics and functional requirements. This improves comfort, functionality, and user satisfaction with prosthetic devices. ML enables robots and prosthetic devices to learn from human interactions and user preferences. Reinforcement learning algorithms, for example, allow robots to adapt their behavior based on feedback, improving collaboration and user satisfaction in assistive scenarios. ML-powered NLP applications facilitate natural communication between users and robotic systems. This includes voice commands for controlling prosthetic devices, receiving feedback, and accessing information, enhancing user experience and accessibility. ML algorithms enable robots to autonomously assist individuals with daily tasks, such as household chores, navigation in public spaces, and remote healthcare monitoring. This promotes independence and improves the quality of life for individuals with disabilities or limited mobility. Implementing ML in robotics and prosthetics requires addressing challenges such as ensuring robustness and safety, mitigating bias in algorithms, optimizing energy efficiency, and integrating seamlessly with human capabilities and environments. As ML techniques continue to advance, the future of robotics and prosthetics holds promise for more intelligent, adaptive, and personalized assistive technologies. These innovations have the potential to redefine mobility and healthcare support for individuals with disabilities, enhancing their autonomy and quality of life.

In summary, ML is driving significant advancements in robotics and prosthetics, empowering individuals with disabilities through enhanced mobility, functionality, and interaction capabilities. These technologies are not only improving physical capabilities but also fostering greater independence and integration into everyday life for users.

7. **ML for Natural Language Processing (NLP) in Healthcare:** ML in NLP is revolutionizing healthcare by enabling the extraction, analysis, and understanding of vast amounts of textual data generated in clinical settings. ML-powered NLP tools parse and analyze unstructured clinical notes, physician narratives, and EHRs. This enables automated extraction of relevant medical information such as diagnoses, treatments, medication history, and patient outcomes, facilitating comprehensive patient care and clinical decision-making. ML algorithms automate medical coding processes by mapping clinical narratives to standardized codes (e.g., International Classification of Diseases (ICD)-10 and Current Procedural Terminology (CPT) codes). This improves accuracy, reduces administrative burden, and ensures compliance with billing regulations, streamlining revenue cycle management in healthcare facilities. ML-enhanced NLP systems provide real-time clinical decision support by integrating patient data from EHRs with medical literature and best practices. These systems assist healthcare providers. ML algorithms extract drug-related information from medical texts, including drug names, dosages, adverse effects, interactions, and prescribing patterns. This supports medication reconciliation, pharmacovigilance, and personalized treatment planning, enhancing patient safety and medication management. ML-powered NLP tools analyze patient feedback from surveys, social media, and online forums to assess patient satisfaction, identify concerns, and detect trends in healthcare service delivery. This information helps healthcare organizations improve patient experience and service quality. ML algorithms match eligible patients to clinical trials based on their medical history, genetic profiles, and demographic data extracted from clinical records. This accelerates recruitment timelines, enhances trial diversity, and improves patient access to experimental treatments. ML-driven search engines and information retrieval systems retrieve relevant medical literature, guidelines, and research articles based on user queries. This supports evidence-based practice, continuing medical education, and research efforts within the healthcare community. ML-powered NLP models [29] monitor and analyze public health data, including news articles, social media posts, and healthcare reports, to detect disease outbreaks, epidemiological trends, and health emergencies in real-time. This early warning system facilitates prompt public health interventions and resource allocation. Robust regulatory frameworks and guidelines ensure the responsible use of NLP technologies to protect patient rights and confidentiality. The future of ML in healthcare NLP includes advancements in conversational AI for patient interaction, multilingual support, integration with wearable devices for real-time data input, and personalized medicine applications. These innovations have the potential to further enhance healthcare delivery, patient outcomes, and population health management.

In conclusion, ML in NLP is transforming healthcare by enabling efficient data analysis, improving clinical decision-making, enhancing patient care quality, and supporting research and public health initiatives.

8. ML for Ethical Considerations: ML in biomedical engineering raises ethical concerns regarding data privacy, bias in algorithms, and the interpretation of AI-driven diagnoses, requiring careful regulation and oversight. In biomedical engineering, ML brings both significant advancements and ethical considerations that must be carefully addressed to ensure responsible development and deployment. Biomedical data, including genetic information, medical records, and imaging data, are highly sensitive. ML systems must employ robust encryption, anonymization techniques, and access controls to protect patient privacy and confidentiality. Compliance with regulations such as the Health Insurance Portability and Accountability Act (HIPAA) is crucial. Biomedical datasets may reflect biases in patient populations, diagnostic practices, or treatment outcomes [30]. ML algorithms trained on biased data can perpetuate disparities in healthcare delivery. Ethical considerations include identifying and mitigating bias in datasets, using fairness-aware algorithms, and ensuring equitable outcomes for diverse patient populations. Obtaining informed consent for data use in biomedical research and ML development is essential. Clear policies on data ownership, sharing, and patient rights regarding data access and withdrawal are necessary. Developers and healthcare providers must ensure transparency in how ML algorithms are developed, validated, and deployed in clinical settings. This includes disclosing algorithmic limitations, explaining decision-making processes to patients and healthcare professionals, and establishing mechanisms for accountability in case of errors or adverse outcomes. ML models in biomedical engineering must undergo rigorous validation to demonstrate safety, efficacy, and reliability before clinical deployment. Adhering to regulatory standards and obtaining appropriate approvals (e.g., Food and Drug Administration (FDA) approval for medical devices) ensures that ML technologies meet quality and safety requirements. ML-driven clinical decision support systems should augment, rather than replace, healthcare professionals' expertise and judgment. Ensuring that algorithms provide understandable explanations and options for human oversight helps maintain healthcare providers' autonomy and responsibility for patient care. ML technologies should aim to improve healthcare accessibility and affordability. Addressing disparities in access to healthcare resources and ensuring equitable distribution of benefits from ML innovations are critical ethical imperatives. Biomedical research using ML should prioritize ethical principles such as beneficence, nonmaleficence, and respect for autonomy. Ethical review boards should oversee research protocols to ensure patient safety, minimize risks, and uphold ethical standards in data collection, analysis, and dissemination. ML technologies developed for biomedical purposes may have dual-use potential, posing ethical dilemmas in terms of unintended consequences or misuse for harmful purposes. Ethical considerations include anticipating potential risks, implementing safeguards, and promoting responsible use to mitigate unintended consequences. Engaging patients, healthcare providers, policymakers, and the public in discussions about the ethical implications of ML in biomedical engineering fosters understanding, trust, and accountability. Education initiatives should raise awareness about the benefits, risks, and ethical considerations associated with emerging technologies.

In conclusion, addressing ethical considerations in ML applications within biomedical engineering requires collaboration among stakeholders, adherence to ethical guidelines and regulations, and a commitment to ensuring patient safety, privacy, fairness, and transparency. By integrating ethical principles into the development and deployment of ML technologies, we can harness their potential to advance healthcare while upholding ethical integrity and societal well-being.

9.5 Opportunities of ML in Biomedical Engineering:

ML offers numerous opportunities to revolutionize biomedical engineering across various domains, enhancing both research capabilities and clinical applications [31–33]. Here are some key opportunities for ML in biomedical engineering:

a. **Personalized Medicine**: ML enables the analysis of large-scale biological and clinical data to tailor medical treatment and interventions according to individual patient characteristics. This includes predicting disease risk, selecting optimal therapies, and optimizing drug dosages based on genetic, environmental, and lifestyle factors (Figure 9.3).

b. **Medical Imaging and Diagnostics**: ML algorithms excel in analyzing complex medical images (e.g., MRI, CT scans, and microscopy images) for automated detection, segmentation, and classification of abnormalities. This improves diagnostic accuracy, speeds up interpretation, and supports early detection of diseases such as cancer and neurological disorders.

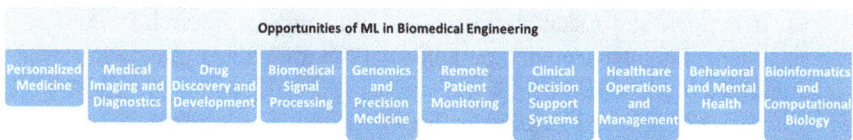

Opportunities of ML in Biomedical Engineering

| Personalized Medicine | Medical Imaging and Diagnostics | Drug Discovery and Development | Biomedical Signal Processing | Genomics and Precision Medicine | Remote Patient Monitoring | Clinical Decision Support Systems | Healthcare Operations and Management | Behavioral and Mental Health | Bioinformatics and Computational Biology |

Figure 9.3   Opportunities of machine learning algorithms in the field of biomedical engineering.

c. **Drug Discovery and Development**: ML accelerates the drug discovery process by predicting molecular interactions, screening large compound libraries, and optimizing lead compounds for efficacy and safety. This reduces the time and cost associated with bringing new drugs to market and enables the discovery of novel therapeutic targets.

d. **Biomedical Signal Processing**: ML techniques enhance the analysis of physiological signals (e.g., ECG, EEG, and EMG) to detect patterns indicative of disease, monitor patient health in real time, and predict clinical outcomes. This supports early intervention and personalized patient management strategies.

e. **Genomics and Precision Medicine**: ML models analyze genomic data to identify genetic variants associated with disease susceptibility, treatment response, and adverse drug reactions. This informs precision medicine approaches by matching patients to targeted therapies and predicting disease progression.

f. **Remote Patient Monitoring**: ML facilitates continuous monitoring of patient health using wearable devices and sensors, capturing data on vital signs, activity levels, and disease biomarkers. This enables early detection of health deterioration, supports chronic disease management, and enhances telemedicine applications.

g. **Clinical Decision Support Systems**: ML-powered decision support systems integrate patient data from EHRs, medical literature, and diagnostic tests to assist healthcare providers in diagnosis, treatment planning, and predicting patient outcomes. This improves clinical decision-making accuracy and efficiency.

h. **Healthcare Operations and Management**: ML optimizes healthcare operations by predicting patient admission rates, optimizing resource allocation (e.g., hospital beds and staffing), and improving workflow efficiency. This enhances healthcare delivery, reduces costs, and enhances patient satisfaction.

i. **Behavioral and Mental Health**: ML models analyze behavioral data (e.g., speech patterns and social media activity) and neurological signals to predict and monitor mental health conditions such as depression, anxiety, and neurodegenerative disorders. This supports early intervention and personalized treatment strategies.

j. **Bioinformatics and Computational Biology**: ML algorithms are integral to analyzing vast amounts of biological data, such as protein sequences, molecular structures, and metabolic pathways. This informs research in areas such as systems biology, drug design, and understanding disease mechanisms at a molecular level.

   i. ML in biomedical engineering presents extensive opportunities to advance healthcare outcomes, from personalized medicine and enhanced diagnostics to drug discovery and healthcare management. By leveraging ML techniques, researchers and healthcare providers can harness the power of data-driven insights to improve patient care, optimize treatments, and accelerate biomedical research.

9.6 Challenges of ML in Biomedical Engineering:

ML in biomedical engineering faces several challenges that must be addressed to ensure its effective and ethical deployment in healthcare and research settings [34, 35] (Figure 9.4). These challenges include:

Data Quality and Quantity: Biomedical datasets are often heterogeneous, noisy, and may have missing values. Ensuring high-quality data collection, curation, and annotation is crucial for training robust ML models. The limited availability of labeled data, especially for rare diseases or specific patient populations, poses additional challenges.

Interpretability and Explainability: ML models, particularly complex ones like deep neural networks, are often considered black boxes, making it difficult to interpret how they arrive at their decisions. In clinical settings, where transparency and trust are critical, explaining model predictions and ensuring interpretability is essential for acceptance and adoption.

Bias and Fairness: Biases present in biomedical data can lead to biased predictions and perpetuate healthcare disparities across demographic groups. Addressing bias through data preprocessing techniques, fairness-aware algorithms, and diverse representation in training datasets is crucial for equitable healthcare outcomes.

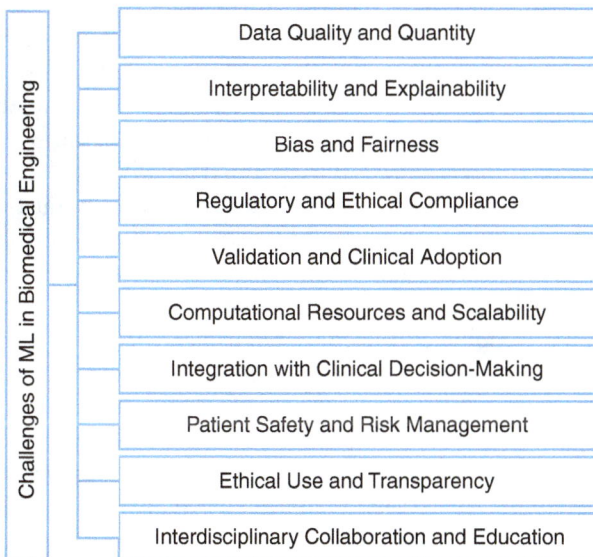

Figure 9.4   Challenges of machine learning algorithms in the field of biomedical engineering.

Regulatory and Ethical Compliance: ML applications in biomedical engineering must comply with stringent regulatory standards (e.g., FDA regulations for medical devices and General Data Protection Regulation (GDPR) for data privacy) to ensure patient safety, data security, and ethical use of AI technologies. Adhering to ethical principles such as informed consent, data anonymization, and protection of patient confidentiality is paramount.

Validation and Clinical Adoption: Validating ML models for clinical use requires rigorous evaluation across diverse patient populations and healthcare settings to demonstrate safety, efficacy, and reliability. Overcoming barriers to adoption, such as integrating ML systems with existing healthcare workflows, gaining clinician trust, and demonstrating real-world impact, is crucial for widespread deployment.

Computational Resources and Scalability: Training and deploying ML models in biomedical applications often require significant computational resources and scalability. Efficient algorithms, cloud computing infrastructure, and collaboration with computational experts are needed to handle large-scale data processing and model optimization.

Integration with Clinical Decision-Making: Integrating ML-driven insights into clinical decision-making workflows without disrupting existing practices or undermining healthcare professionals' expertise poses a challenge. Ensuring that ML algorithms complement rather than replace human judgment and providing actionable recommendations that align with clinical guidelines are essential considerations.

Patient Safety and Risk Management: ML models must prioritize patient safety by minimizing risks such as erroneous diagnoses, incorrect treatment recommendations, or adverse reactions to medications. Robust risk management strategies, continuous monitoring of model performance, and implementing fail-safe mechanisms are critical to mitigate potential harm.

Ethical Use and Transparency: Ensuring ethical use of ML technologies involves addressing concerns related to unintended consequences, dual-use risks, and societal impact. Transparency in how data is collected, used, and shared, along with fostering public awareness and engagement, helps build trust and accountability in AI-driven biomedical applications.

Interdisciplinary Collaboration and Education: Bridging the gap between biomedical researchers, data scientists, clinicians, and policymakers through interdisciplinary collaboration and education is essential for overcoming technical, regulatory, and ethical challenges. Promoting a shared understanding of ML capabilities, limitations, and best practices fosters responsible innovation and effective implementation in biomedical engineering.

Addressing the challenges of ML in biomedical engineering requires a concerted effort from stakeholders across disciplines to ensure that AI technologies contribute to improving healthcare outcomes while upholding ethical standards, patient safety, and regulatory compliance. By tackling these challenges, ML has the potential to revolutionize biomedical research, clinical practice, and healthcare delivery for the benefit of patients worldwide.

9.7 Future Enhancements of ML in Biomedical Engineering

The future of ML in biomedical engineering holds tremendous potential for advancing healthcare through innovative technologies and methodologies [36, 37]. Here are some key areas where future enhancements in ML are expected:

1. **Interpretability and Explainability**: Developing ML models that are more interpretable and capable of explaining their decisions will be crucial for gaining trust and acceptance in clinical settings. Techniques such as model distillation, attention mechanisms, and generating human-understandable explanations (e.g., using NLP) will be explored to enhance interpretability.
2. **Multi-modal Data Integration**: Integrating diverse data sources including genomic data, medical images, EHRs, wearable sensor data, and patient-reported outcomes will enable comprehensive patient profiling and personalized medicine. ML techniques like multimodal fusion, transfer learning, and federated learning will facilitate effective integration and analysis of heterogeneous data types.
3. **Continuous Learning and Adaptive Systems**: Developing ML algorithms that can continuously learn from new data and adapt to evolving patient conditions and treatment outcomes will support dynamic and personalized healthcare interventions. Techniques such as online learning, reinforcement learning, and adaptive algorithms will enable models to improve over time and adjust to changing healthcare needs.
4. **Robustness and Security**: Enhancing the robustness of ML models against adversarial attacks and ensuring data security and privacy will be critical for deploying AI technologies in healthcare. The research will focus on developing robust training techniques, anomaly detection methods, and privacy-preserving algorithms (e.g., differential privacy) to safeguard sensitive biomedical data.
5. **Biomedical Image Analysis**: Advancements in ML algorithms for medical imaging will focus on improving accuracy, speed, and reliability in tasks such as image segmentation, feature extraction, and disease classification. Deep learning architectures tailored for medical image analysis, along with techniques for domain adaptation and transfer learning, will enable the effective utilization of large-scale image datasets.
6. **Clinical Decision Support Systems**: Enhancing ML-driven decision support systems to provide real-time, actionable insights for healthcare professionals will optimize clinical workflows and improve patient outcomes. Integration

with EHRs, predictive analytics for risk stratification, and automated treatment recommendations will facilitate evidence-based medicine and personalized patient care.

7. **Natural Language Processing (NLP) in Healthcare**: Advancements in NLP will enable automated extraction, summarization, and analysis of clinical notes, biomedical literature, and patient records. ML models for clinical coding, sentiment analysis of patient feedback, and information retrieval will streamline healthcare operations and enhance understanding of healthcare data.

8. **AI-driven Drug Discovery and Development**: ML will continue to play a pivotal role in accelerating drug discovery pipelines by predicting drug-target interactions, optimizing lead compounds, and identifying potential therapeutic candidates. Integration of ML with high-throughput screening technologies, molecular simulations, and virtual drug screening approaches will expedite the development of novel treatments for complex diseases.

9. **Ethical AI Governance and Regulation**: Establishing robust ethical guidelines, governance frameworks, and regulatory policies specific to AI in biomedical engineering will ensure responsible development, deployment, and use of ML technologies. Collaborative efforts among policymakers, industry stakeholders, and healthcare professionals will promote transparency, fairness, and accountability in AI-driven healthcare innovations.

10. **Collaborative Research and Open Science**: Encouraging collaboration among researchers, fostering open access to biomedical datasets, and promoting reproducibility of ML studies will accelerate scientific discovery and innovation in biomedical engineering. Platforms for sharing data, code, and pretrained models, along with initiatives for crowdsourcing AI solutions to healthcare challenges, will drive collective efforts toward transformative advancements in healthcare.

Future enhancements in ML for biomedical engineering will focus on developing interpretable and adaptive AI systems, integrating diverse data sources for personalized medicine, ensuring robustness and security, and fostering ethical AI governance. These advancements have the potential to revolutionize healthcare delivery, improve patient outcomes, and enable precision medicine tailored to individual patient needs.

9.8 Conclusion

In conclusion, the integration of ML in biomedical engineering represents a transformative frontier with profound implications. By leveraging vast datasets and advanced algorithms, ML techniques enable unprecedented insights into complex biological processes, disease mechanisms, and personalized treatment strategies. The synergy between computational power and biomedical expertise holds promise for accelerating medical innovation, enhancing diagnostic accuracy, and optimizing therapeutic outcomes. However, challenges such as data quality, interpretability, and ethical considerations underscore the need for continued interdisciplinary collaboration and rigorous validation. As we navigate this evolving landscape, embracing the potential of ML in biomedical engineering with a balanced approach will be crucial to unlocking its full potential for improving global health outcomes.

References

[1] D. Huang, E. A. Swanson, *et al.*, "Optical Coherence Tomography," *Science*, vol. 254, no. 5035, pp. 1178–1181, 1991.

[2] B. He *et al.*, "Grand Challenges in Interfacing Engineering with Life Sciences and Medicine," in *IEEE Transactions on Biomedical Engineering*, vol. 60, no. 3, pp. 589–598, March 2013, doi: 10.1109/TBME.2013.2244886

[3] A. Trnčić, D. M. Ajayi, E. Hodžić, L. Spahić Bećirović, L. Gurbeta Pokvić and A. Badnjević, "Biomedical Signal Analysis for Automatic Detection of Diseases and Disorders in Prenatal Age," *2022 11th Mediterranean Conference on Embedded Computing (MECO)*, Budva, Montenegro, 2022, pp. 1–4, doi: 10.1109/MECO55406. 2022.9797105

[4] S. Dixit, A. Gaikwad, V. Vyas, M. Shindikar and K. Kamble, "United Neurological Study of Disorders: Alzheimer's Disease, Parkinson's Disease Detection, Anxiety Detection, and Stress Detection Using Various Machine Learning Algorithms," *2022 International Conference on Signal and Information Processing (IConSIP)*, Pune, India, 2022, pp. 1–6, doi: 10.1109/IConSIP49665.2022.10007434

[5] K. Grifantini, "Electrical Stimulation: A Panacea for Disease?: DARPA Investigates New Bioelectrical Interfaces for a Range of Disorders," *IEEE Pulse*, vol. 7, no. 4, pp. 30–35, July-Aug. 2016, doi: 10.1109/MPUL.2016.2563838

[6] B. He *et al.*, "Grand Challenges in Interfacing Engineering with Life Sciences and Medicine," in *IEEE Transactions on Biomedical Engineering*, vol. 60, no. 3, pp. 589–598, March 2013, doi: 10.1109/TBME.2013.2244886

[7] S. Dixit, A. Gaikwad, V. Vyas, M. Shindikar and K. Kamble, "United Neurological Study of Disorders: Alzheimer's Disease, Parkinson's Disease Detection, Anxiety Detection, and Stress Detection Using Various Machine Learning Algorithms," *2022 International Conference on Signal and Information Processing (IConSIP)*, Pune, India, 2022, pp. 1–6, doi: 10.1109/IConSIP49665.2022.10007434

[8] A. Trnčić, D. M. Ajayi, E. Hodžić, L. Spahić Bećirović, L. Gurbeta Pokvić and A. Badnjević, "Biomedical Signal Analysis for Automatic Detection of Diseases and Disorders in Prenatal Age," *2022 11th Mediterranean Conference on Embedded Computing (MECO)*, Budva, Montenegro, 2022, pp. 1–4, doi: 10.1109/MECO55406. 2022.9797105

[9] B. Peng *et al.*, "Computer Aided Analysis of Cognitive Disorder in Patients with Parkinsonism Using Machine Learning Method with Multilevel ROI-Based Features," *2016 9th International Congress on Image and Signal Processing, BioMedical Engineering and Informatics (CISP-BMEI)*, Datong, China, 2016, pp. 1792–1796, doi: 10.1109/ CISP-BMEI.2016.7853008

[10] E. S. Emamian and A. Abdi, "Complex Human Disorders and Molecular System Engineering: Historical Perspective and Potential Impacts," *2009 Annual International Conference of the IEEE Engineering in Medicine and Biology Society*, Minneapolis, MN, 2009, pp. 1083–1085, doi: 10.1109/IEMBS.2009.5334895

[11] P. Chalacheva and M. C. K. Khoo, "Integrating Machine Learning with Biomedical Signal Processing and Systems Analysis: An Applications-based Course," *2023 45th Annual International Conference of the IEEE Engineering in Medicine & Biology Society (EMBC)*, Sydney, Australia, 2023, pp. 1–4, doi: 10.1109/EMBC40787.2023.10340498

[12] K. Tsarapatsani *et al.*, "Machine Learning Models for Cardiovascular Disease Events Prediction," *2022 44th Annual International Conference of the IEEE Engineering in Medicine & Biology Society (EMBC)*, Glasgow, Scotland, UK, 2022, pp. 1066–1069, doi: 10.1109/EMBC48229.2022.9871121

[13] S. N. Mohammed, M. Serdar Guzel and E. Bostanci, "Classification and Success Investigation of Biomedical Data Sets Using Supervised Machine Learning Models," *2019 3rd International Symposium on Multidisciplinary Studies and Innovative Technologies (ISMSIT)*, Ankara, Turkey, 2019, pp. 1–5, doi: 10.1109/ISMSIT.2019.8932734

[14] İ. B. Aydilek, "Examining Effects of the Support Vector Machines Kernel Types on Biomedical Data Classification," *2018 International Conference on Artificial Intelligence and Data Processing (IDAP)*, Malatya, Turkey, 2018, pp. 1–4, doi: 10.1109/IDAP.2018.8620879

[15] W. Kim and J. Seok, "Privacy-Preserving Collaborative Machine Learning in Biomedical Applications," *2022 International Conference on Artificial Intelligence in Information and Communication (ICAIIC)*, Korea, Republic of Jeju Island, 2022, pp. 179–183, doi: 10.1109/ICAIIC54071.2022.9722703

[16] C. A. Flores and R. Verschae, "A Generic Semi-Supervised and Active Learning Framework for Biomedical Text Classification," *2022 44th Annual International Conference of the IEEE Engineering in Medicine & Biology Society (EMBC)*, Glasgow, Scotland, UK, 2022, pp. 4445–4448, doi: 10.1109/EMBC48229.2022.9871846

[17] K. M. Jaeger *et al.*, "Machine Learning-based Detection of In-Utero Fetal Presentation from Non-Invasive Fetal ECG," *2022 IEEE-EMBS International Conference on Biomedical and Health Informatics (BHI)*, Ioannina, Greece, 2022, pp. 01–04, doi: 10.1109/BHI56158.2022.9926804

[18] M. M. Mishu, "A Patient Oriented Framework using Big Data & C-means Clustering for Biomedical Engineering Applications," *2019 International Conference on Robotics, Electrical and Signal Processing Techniques (ICREST)*, Dhaka, Bangladesh, 2019, pp. 113–115, doi: 10.1109/ICREST.2019.8644276

[19] E. A. Bayrak, P. Kırcı and T. Ensari, "Comparison of Machine Learning Methods for Breast Cancer Diagnosis," *2019 Scientific Meeting on Electrical-Electronics & Biomedical Engineering and Computer Science (EBBT)*, Istanbul, Turkey, 2019, pp. 1–3, doi: 10.1109/EBBT.2019.8741990

[20] R. Pinky, S. J. Singh and C. Pankaj, "Human Activities Recognition and Monitoring System Using Machine Learning Techniques," *2022 Trends in Electrical, Electronics, Computer Engineering Conference (TEECCON)*, Bengaluru, India, 2022, pp. 62–66, doi: 10.1109/TEECCON54414.2022.9854829

[21] H. Sami, M. Sagheer, K. Riaz, M. Q. Mehmood and M. Zubair, "Machine Learning-Based Approaches For Breast Cancer Detection in Microwave Imaging," *2021 IEEE USNC-URSI Radio Science Meeting (Joint with AP-S Symposium)*, Singapore, 2021, pp. 72–73, doi: 10.23919/USNC-URSI51813.2021.9703518

[22] K. Zhao and H. -C. So, "Drug Repositioning for Schizophrenia and Depression/Anxiety Disorders: A Machine Learning Approach Leveraging Expression Data," *IEEE Journal of Biomedical and Health Informatics*, vol. 23, no. 3, pp. 1304–1315, May 2019, doi: 10.1109/JBHI.2018.2856535

[23] A. Suganthi, N. Sarmiladevi, A. Indhuja, and G. Venkatesan, "Performance Analysis of Machine Learning Classification for Parkinson's Disease from Biomedical Audio Data," *2023 Intelligent Computing and Control for Engineering and Business Systems (ICCEBS)*, Chennai, India, 2023, pp. 1–5, doi: 10.1109/ICCEBS58601.2023.10448605

[24] C. Bunterngchit and Y. Bunterngchit, "A Comparative Study of Machine Learning Models for Parkinson's Disease Detection," *2022 International Conference on Decision Aid Sciences and Applications (DASA)*, Chiangrai, Thailand, 2022, pp. 465–469, doi: 10.1109/DASA54658.2022.9765159

[25] M. -P. Hosseini, A. Hosseini and K. Ahi, "A Review on Machine Learning for EEG Signal Processing in Bioengineering," *IEEE Reviews in Biomedical Engineering*, vol. 14, pp. 204–218, 2021, doi: 10.1109/RBME.2020.2969915

[26] D. Maheshwari, B. Garcia-Zapirain and D. Sierra-Sosa, "Quantum Machine Learning Applications in the Biomedical Domain: A Systematic Review," *IEEE Access*, vol. 10, pp. 80463–80484, 2022, doi: 10.1109/ACCESS.2022.3195044

[27] H. Chang, J. Han, C. Zhong, A. M. Snijders and J. -H. Mao, "Unsupervised Transfer Learning via Multi-Scale Convolutional Sparse Coding for Biomedical Applications," *IEEE Transactions on Pattern Analysis and Machine Intelligence*, vol. 40, no. 5, pp. 1182–1194, 1 May 2018, doi: 10.1109/TPAMI.2017.2656884

[28] A. Anastasiou, S. Pitoglou, T. Androutsou, E. Kostalas, G. Matsopoulos and D. Koutsouris, "MODELHealth: An Innovative Software Platform for Machine Learning in Healthcare Leveraging Indoor Localization Services," *2019 20th IEEE International Conference on Mobile Data Management (MDM)*, Hong Kong, China, 2019, pp. 443–446, doi: 10.1109/MDM.2019.000-5

[29] L. Vorberg *et al.*, "Prediction of Stress Coping Capabilities from Nightly Heart Rate Patterns using Machine Learning," *2023 IEEE EMBS International Conference on Biomedical and Health Informatics (BHI)*, Pittsburgh, PA, 2023, pp. 1–4, doi: 10.1109/BHI58575.2023.10313401

[30] A. Shrivastava, M. Chakkaravathy and M. A. Shah, "A Comprehensive Analysis of Machine Learning Techniques in Biomedical Image Processing Using Convolutional Neural Network," *2022 5th International Conference on Contemporary Computing and Informatics (IC3I)*, Uttar Pradesh, India, 2022, pp. 1363–1369, doi: 10.1109/IC3I56241.2022.10072911

[31] L. Rettenberger, M. Schilling, S. Elser, M. Böhland and M. Reischl, "Self-Supervised Learning for Annotation Efficient Biomedical Image Segmentation," *IEEE Transactions on Biomedical Engineering*, vol. 70, no. 9, pp. 2519–2528, Sept. 2023, doi: 10.1109/TBME.2023.3252889

[32] S. Briouza, H. Gritli, N. Khraief, S. Belghith and D. Singh, "EMG Signal Classification for Human Hand Rehabilitation via Two Machine Learning Techniques: kNN and SVM," *2022 5th International Conference on Advanced Systems and Emergent Technologies (IC_ASET)*, Hammamet, Tunisia, 2022, pp. 412–417, doi: 10.1109/ IC_ASET53395.2022.9765856

[33] J. Berman, R. Hinson, I. -C. Lee and H. Huang, "Harnessing Machine Learning and Physiological Knowledge for a Novel EMG-Based Neural-Machine Interface," *IEEE Transactions on Biomedical Engineering*, vol. 70, no. 4, pp. 1125–1136, April 2023, doi: 10.1109/TBME.2022.3210892

[34] R. Rajkumar, L. N. Vempaty, R. Thiyagarajan, C. Kavida, and H. Hemane, "Enhancing Biomedical Image Interpretation Through a Hybrid Machine Learning Algorithm," *2023 7th International Conference on Electronics, Communication and Aerospace Technology (ICECA)*, Coimbatore, India, 2023, pp. 1126–1131, doi: 10.1109/ ICECA58529.2023.10395806

[35] S. Turgut, M. Dağtekin and T. Ensari, "Microarray Breast Cancer Data Classification Using Machine Learning Methods," *2018 Electric Electronics, Computer Science, Biomedical Engineerings' Meeting (EBBT)*, Istanbul, Turkey, 2018, pp. 1–3, doi: 10.1109/EBBT.2018.8391468

[36] M. Bahrami and M. Forouzanfar, "Sleep Apnea Detection from Single-Lead ECG: A Comprehensive Analysis of Machine Learning and Deep Learning Algorithms," *IEEE Transactions on Instrumentation and Measurement*, vol. 71, pp. 1–11, 2022, 4003011, doi: 10.1109/TIM.2022.3151947

[37] M. Li *et al.*, "Machine Learning in Electromagnetics with Applications to Biomedical Imaging: A Review," *IEEE Antennas and Propagation Magazine*, vol. 63, no. 3, pp. 39–51, June 2021, doi: 10.1109/MAP.2020.3043469

Chapter 10

Intelligent Tools and Techniques for Real-Life Diseases

Pradeep Singh Rawat, Prateek Kumar Soni and Punit Gupta

10.1 Introduction

The management of diseases such as cancer, cardiovascular disease (CVD), neuro-logical disorders, diabetes, tuberculosis, and sepsis was highly difficult before the development of Artificial Intelligence (AI) because of the shortcomings in conventional diagnostic and treatment techniques. These diseases posed significant obstacles in healthcare, often leading to delayed diagnoses, inadequate treatment plans, and poor patient outcomes. Since then, AI has started to revolutionize these fields by enabling more precise diagnosis, individualized treatment plans, and enhanced management techniques, giving millions of patients suffering from these illnesses hope.

Cancer has always been a daunting disease to diagnose and treat, primarily due to its complex nature and the diversity of its forms. Previously, radiologists and physicians manually interpreted results from medical imaging procedures such as CT scans, MRIs, and X-rays to diagnose cancer. Human error was a common occurrence in this procedure, which often resulted in late-stage detections when treatment options became limited and less effective. Additionally, many patients were given generic treatment regimens that neglected to take into account their unique cancer profiles due to the lack of precision in detecting particular genetic mutations and cancer biomarkers. AI is now starting to completely transform the medical field by using machine learning (ML) algorithms to enhance image analysis, increasing the

DOI: 10.1201/9781003617013-10

precision of early detection, and making it a lot easier to create customized treatment plans based on a patient's genetic makeup.

Heart attacks, strokes, and heart failure are examples of CVDs, which have long been the world's leading cause of death. One of the primary challenges in managing CVDs was the lack of robust diagnostic and prognostic tools capable of predicting cardiac events. Conventional techniques such as electrocardiograms (ECGs) and blood pressure monitoring produced limited data, often failing to detect early signs or assess individual risk accurately. Now, this landscape has changed due to AI's predictive analytics capabilities, which analyze patient data to find patterns and correlations that point to the risk of cardiovascular events. This development greatly improves patient outcomes and lowers mortality rates by allowing healthcare providers to intervene earlier with customized preventive measures.

It was indeed tough to monitor diseases such as Alzheimer's and Parkinson's. Such diseases are progressive in nature with subtle early warning signs. Therefore, it was indeed next to impossible to treat these diseases well because the diseases were often discovered when serious damage to neurological activity had already occurred. The traditional diagnostic method utilized mostly clinical observations and cognitive evaluation that lacked the ability to detect subtle changes in the brain. With the development of AI technologies, especially the ML and recognition algorithms related to the analysis of brain scans and other neurological data, possibilities for early indicators have emerged. In addition to better treatment, early diagnosis provides more effective plans as well as alleviates disease progressions, thus enhancing quality of life.

Diabetes management was mainly based on spot glucose monitoring and standardized protocols of treatment; this generally resulted in the patient being left with suboptimal blood sugar control. The lack of real-time data made it relatively difficult to predict fluctuations in glucose levels, leaving the patient vulnerable to episodes of hypoglycemia or hyperglycemia. AI has greatly improved this field as it uses the data that continuous glucose monitoring gives forth to predict trends in blood sugar levels and even suggest accurate dosing of insulin. Real-time analysis in such cases has enabled more individualized management of diabetes and reduction of complications while patients who have diabetes live better.

Other infectious diseases, for example, tuberculosis and sepsis, have for long times been challenging to diagnose accurately. Tuberculosis used to be detected traditionally by sputum tests and chest X-rays whose sensitivity and specificity in early onset identification of the disease is very low. For sepsis, detection or diagnosis should have been prompt and accurate because the delay in detection led to organ failure most of the time. AI technologies have further led to the development of better diagnostic apparatuses, which can scan a large amount of clinical data in real-time for quick and accurate detection of disease. Quicker intervention is necessary to prevent sometimes grave consequences of infectious diseases.

This chapter will elaborate on these diseases by taking a transformative role of AI in overcoming historical challenges: revolutions in the detection, diagnosis, and management of such conditions-precise, personalized, and efficient healthcare.

10.2 AI-Powered Diagnostic Systems

AI-driven diagnostic systems are revolutions in the medical world concerning the precision, speed, and efficiency of disease detection and diagnosis. With advanced algorithms, ML, and deep learning, it is now possible to automatically scan enormous volumes of medical data for specific patterns related to health conditions, which in turn offers support for clinical decision-making. Its key applications are in medical imaging, predictive analytics, pathology, and personalized medicine. Several diagnostics based on AI have already impacted the healthcare systems remarkably, revolutionizing how diseases should be diagnosed and treated.

IBM Watson: IBM Watson for Oncology is a cognitive computing service, which provides an AI-based diagnostic system that helps oncologists make the right decisions regarding treatment choices for patients. Trained with millions of medical literature sources and data from clinical trials and patient records, Watson may analyze the health data of a patient and make corresponding recommendations on various types of cancer for personalized treatment options. IBM Watson considers a number of factors to be taken into account, including medical history, genetic profiles, and current patient conditions, to give recommendations for the most effective therapies. As a result of IBM Watson's capability to process huge volumes of data and quickly analyze them, oncologists can develop treatment plans that are far more acutely tailored to individual needs [1].

Google DeepMind Health: Another example of AI diagnostic technology developed for diagnosing medical images and applying predictive analytics is Google's DeepMind Health. Notable among its achievements in its work is in the ophthalmological sphere: it teamed up with Moorfields Eye Hospital in London to develop an AI system that can identify AMD and diabetic retinopathy from retinal scans. The AI algorithm can identify all the early signs of these conditions and do so with a level of precision that is comparable to what an expert ophthalmologist would produce. Early diagnosis and subsequent treatment will help this technology from DeepMind prevent worse vision loss in patients suffering from such conditions [2].

Aidoc: Aidoc is an AI-powered diagnostic system and has particularly been designed to analyze medical imaging, particularly radiology. Aiding deep learning algorithms and analyses of CT scans, MRIs, and X-rays for seeing critical conditions such as hemorrhages in the brain, strokes, pulmonary embolisms, and fractures, the system has been designed into the radiology department's existing workflows. It provides real-time alerts to the attention of the radiologists in case abnormalities appear within the scans. Such early identification of emergency cases enables the health care provider to place a priority on taking proper care of the patient and thus provides an opportunity for treatment initiation to occur earlier in the course of the emergency case.

Aidoc's AI-based technology has been used to greatly help in reducing errors in diagnoses and hence helped improve the outcomes of patients in the radiology departments [3].

Zebra Medical Vision: Zebra Medical Vision has designed analysis tools based on AI applied to numerous different health conditions, including liver disease, CVD, issues in regard to bone density, and breast cancer. Its algorithms scan millions of medical images to recognize patterns and anomalies potentially indicating the onset of these diseases. The technology of Zebra Medical Vision works hand in hand with radiologists, as AI-driven insights assist in the early detection of disease and monitoring. The company has set out to provide high-quality diagnostics, particularly to regions with a deficit in the availability of medical professionals [4].

10.3 Wearable Health Devices and Mobile Applications

Wearable health devices and smart mobile applications have become extremely integral components of contemporary healthcare, bringing together technology and personalized health management. The tools enable constant monitoring of health conditions, tracking of fitness goals, and chronic diseases, done with unprecedented ease and precision. Therefore, devices such as smartwatches, fitness trackers, and specialized medical wearables coupled with health-centric mobile apps provide seamless ways of collecting and later crunching health data. Technologies like heartbeats and blood pressure to monitor the patterns in sleeping, physical activity, as well as mental well-being allow the user to gain such clear knowledge about their health. The raw data becomes actionable information for both the health device wearers and mobile applications in connection with proactive healthcare as citizens are educated to take control of wellness and ensure conscious lifestyle choices. It seems this innovation determines the future of the reshaping of the preventive care landscape and that of personalized medicine.

10.3.1 Role of Wearables in Health Monitoring

Integration of AI with wearable technologies has been highly effective in the healthcare industry, including allowing for continuous monitoring of health, better patient results, and proactive personal well-being. With wearables fitness trackers, smartwatches, and medical-grade wearables, people can monitor all their health metrics, including heart rate, sleep patterns, physical activity, and some specific medical conditions, through robust sensor technology and data analytics that implement AI methods. Continuous real-time monitoring from devices such as the Apple Watch, Fitbit, and Garmin enables people to discover changes in their health such as arrhythmias which may signal a rhythm disorder such as atrial fibrillation and lead to early treatment. This enables patients to manage chronic diseases such as diabetes and cardiovascular conditions by giving them all the insights of real-time data analysis in order to take precise treatment measures. As such constant feedback enhances their health-related decision-making skills, these also enhance the management of diseases and the quality of life. For example, wearables, such as Omron HeartGuide, have functions that enable blood pressure monitoring [5]. Devices that track patterns when sleeping help diagnose sleep apnea and then correlate it with wider health problems such as heart disease. The integration of such wearables into the healthcare system would allow for remote patient monitoring; thus, the doctor would be able to receive real-time data and make informed clinical judgments without frequent visits to the physical facility. Such fluid data integration allows for tailored care, enhanced diagnostic precision, and fine-tuned treatment plans, especially for patients who have chronic diseases or are recovering from an operation. Though technical issues such as the number of inaccuracies in reporting data, confidentiality issues, and adherence among users are the major challenges being encountered, continued technological advancement is enhancing the credibility and safety of wearables, making them inevitable in the health sector of today [6].

10.3.2 Mobile Apps for Disease Management

The management of patient conditions and interaction with healthcare providers in disease management uses of mobile applications have made it possible for patients to change the way they monitor their conditions and follow treatment plans. For example, among such apps, there is convenience in a person being able to track symptoms and manage medication schedules, monitor his vital signs, and even receive personalized health recommendations. In chronic diseases that include diabetes, hypertension, asthma, and mental disorders, mobile applications can offer real-time insight and reminders to help patients stay on top of treatment regimens.

> **MySugr**: An application specifically designed for diabetes management. MySugr users can log blood sugar levels, monitor what they are eating, and record their doses of insulin. The application provides feedback and analysis so that the patient can better understand what he or she is doing and make informed decisions regarding health. Another famous application is Medisafe. It generally focuses on medication management. Medisafe helps a patient set up a medication schedule, receives reminders for his dosages, and tracks adherence. The app would remind a user to take the medicine, in case the user has missed a dose. In this way, medication compliance would improve and the complications related to missing medications would be reduced [7].
>
> **Va FitHeart**: An example would be to have an app for tracking heart health or management of heart-related conditions, through daily tips and reminders of

medication intake, and education concerning lifestyle changes. It helps monitor the levels of blood pressure and cholesterol, as well as physical activity levels, making it easy to manage heart-related conditions. The other example is **AsthmaMD**, for people suffering from asthma, as it tracks symptoms, medication use, and peak flow measurements. The app produces reports sent to the healthcare providers leading to better communication and ultimately a tailored treatment plan for the individual.[8, 9]

HeadSpace and Calm: Applications such as Calm and Headspace give guided meditations, breathing practices, and mindfulness training to address stress and anxiety in mental health. Such applications benefit mental well-being, giving mechanisms for dealing with oneself, which would be incredibly useful for those afflicted by mental health disorders. In deeper conditions of mental health, the mobile application **Talkspace** brings teletherapy services by linking the user with a licensed therapist through messaging or video calls, making it a tablelot easier to reach access to mental care [10, 11].

In addition, these mobile applications also enable other telemedicine care-related features that entail users receiving consultations with a professional healthcare provider while saving physical time by reducing visits to a clinic. On the analytics side, through AI, such apps can make insightful predictions toward proactive disease flare or complication prevention. With the advancement of mobile technology, apps have become unavailable and indispensable in managing chronic diseases in order to achieve better health outcomes and empowerment of the patient with real-time data and professional guidance at their fingertips.

10.4 NLP in Healthcare

Natural Language Processing (NLP) is one of the basic transformative technologies applied on the healthcare side, greatly improving how healthcare professionals access and process large amounts of clinical data. Human language analysis algorithms enable NLP to enable providers of health care to tease out meaningful information that might lie in unstructured data such as clinical notes, patient records, and even medical literature. This is specifically very critical in a field where the timeliness and accuracy of information are translated into better patient outcomes and effective care strategies.

One of the primary applications of NLP is EHR analysis. The huge amount of information contained in EHRs includes clinical notes, histories of medications, and diagnostic data. However, much of this data is unstructured and not amenable to analysis through traditional means. NLP algorithms can process these records, thereby discovering key concepts, relationships, and patterns that might otherwise go unnoticed. Through the process of transforming unstructured data into well-structured forms, NLP enables healthcare professionals to gain insights that help in making clinical decisions, delivering good care to the patients, and further administrative efficiencies.

Besides such capability in EHRs, NLP plays an even greater role in clinical documentation. Healthcare providers spend long hours documenting patient encounters, which by itself takes time away from patients. Clinical conversations can be recorded and formatted in real time using NLP tools to automate them. More than productivity, this automation will ensure that all pertinent information about patients is captured correctly and with detail. Another area where NLP can be applied is standardizing documentation practices across different healthcare systems, which leads to better communication and data sharing among providers.

Finally, NLP plays a very important role in clinical research by simplifying literature review processes and data extraction procedures. With the aid of NLP algorithms, researchers can go through massive databases of medical literature and identify relevant studies, extract key findings, and, above all, summarize lots of information very efficiently. Its worth, therefore, was most apparently placed in areas such as oncology and pharmacology, where the volume of published research is almost overwhelming, and keeping abreast of the latest findings means that truly informed decisions can be made. NLP reduced the burden that researchers have in sifting through their literature reviews by allowing them to save time for critical analysis and hypothesis generation.

In the healthcare sector, NLP is changing the way professionals have access to and interact with clinical data, and subsequently, patient care, research efficiency, and public health response will become better. The increasing number of potential applications of NLP in healthcare will be countless as the technology becomes more sophisticated, opening new avenues to enhance the quality and efficiency of care delivery.

10.4.1 Virtual Assistants and Chatbots in Patient Interaction

Babylon Health Chatbot: Babylon offers a chatbot that gives health assessments to users based on the symptoms they experience. Patients could answer a series of questions about how they feel, and possible conditions would be reported along with an indication of whether patients might need additional advice from a health professional. The app also integrates telemedicine services, so users can gain access to consultations with healthcare professionals directly through the platform [12].

Woebot: Woebot is an app that comes in the form of a chatbot that provides emotional support via cognitive-behavioral therapy techniques. One can vent their feelings to the chatbot, and with guidance and strategies, one will receive help to ensure anxiety and depression are put in check. Therefore, the AI virtual assistant bridges this gap by offering confidential access to those seeking mental health support [13].

10.5 Computer Vision Tools

The computer vision tool has revolutionized the health landscape. It now allows for the analysis and interpretation of medical images with accuracy and efficiency hitherto unattained. Advanced algorithms and ML techniques help the healthcare professional diagnose diseases, monitor progress in treatment, and predict patient outcomes from visual data. Applications of computer vision are found in practically every area of health care, from radiology and pathology to dermatology, where it scans X-rays, MRIs, CT scans, and even skin lesions. This allows automatic anomaly detection, quantification of features, and real-time feedback to enhance the diagnostic capabilities of providers in health care in terms of faster intervention with higher accuracy. This integration also includes how technology in computer vision evolves with AI and big data analytics to further heighten its impact on patient care and workflow improvements but may eventually even improve health outcomes.

10.5.1 AI-based Image Processing for Diagnosis

With the Internet of Things (IoT) and AI, the image processing of medical diagnosis is revolutionized in the sense that it is more accurate and quicker than any other test used in the medical field-from x-rays to MRIs, CT scans, and ultrasounds. With accuracy, these technologies analyze images, detect patterns and anomalies, and categorize conditions using sophisticated algorithms and deep learning methods. AI techniques, for instance, can distinguish between the signs of pneumonia, nodules, and fractures in radiology. This leads to a significant reduction in the chance of missed diagnoses and faster turnaround times, particularly in emergency situations.

In oncology, AI assists in tumor detection and characterization, such as breast cancer diagnosis using images from mammograms, so fewer false positives and fewer unnecessary biopsies are conducted. In dermatology, AI-driven apps examine skin lesions for symptoms of skin cancer, and the application recommends when to refer to professional evaluation. Additionally, dynamic imaging is enhanced further with AI in areas such as echocardiography where, automatically, cardiac structures are measured and abnormalities identified. Although the future of AI looks promising in image processing by introducing higher accuracy diagnostics, greater patient outcomes, and revolutionizing care through proactive data-driven techniques for detection and management, its usage is riddled with key challenges including privacy issues over data and algorithmic transparency.

AI in Oncology: AI in this field goes a long way. It has helped greatly in diagnosis, planning the treatment process of patients with cancer, and managing them. AI algorithms analyze large datasets, including images in medicine and genomic data, besides electronic health records (EHRs), to identify specific patterns and predict outcomes that, in turn, help oncologists in making decisions. AI has truly found fertile ground in medical imaging: using algorithms to locate tumors within radiology scans that achieve almost the same accuracy rate as human experts and significantly decrease the rate of both false positives and false negatives. It allows for personalized medicine; genomic data is analyzed for the presence of particular mutations and the identification of biomarkers in tumors. This information enables oncologists to treat patients matched by the patient's profile of cancer, thereby maximizing the effectiveness of therapy while minimizing side effects. NLP technologies are also important for extracting patient's clinical information from unstructured clinical notes in order to keep oncologists up to date with recent research and treatment guidelines. With AI-driven decision-support systems implemented into clinical workflows, oncologists can get evidence-based recommendations and risk assessments. Integration of AI in oncology may be a step toward better patient outcomes, streamlined processes, and ultimately, good quality cancer care [14].

AI in Dermatology: The applications of AI in dermatology also include early melanoma and other types of skin cancer detection. With a mobile application powered by AI, the user would simply take photographs of moles or skin lesions, and further analysis by an algorithm would then determine their probability of malignancy. Such advice empowers patients to be early for professional diagnosis and proceed with treatment, thus avoiding poor outcomes.

Next, AI is being used to simplify clinical workflows such that it will enable dermatologists to prioritize some cases at the expense of others depending on urgency and which of the treatments available to pursue. The use of NLP technologies in documentation improves the process since the relevant information extracted from clinical notes can automatically be included. In dermatology, the potential role of AI is also expected to grow with more advanced diagnostic accuracy, personalized treatment plans, and interactive patient engagement in their healthcare [15].

AI in echocardiography - AI-based algorithms, including deep learning, automatically define the anomalies in cardiac structures, which include ventricles, atria, and valves, from echocardiographic images. Automated analysis cuts hours spent on analysis and reduces inter-operator variability based on consistent and reliable assessments. For instance, with AI measurement, ejection fraction, wall motion abnormalities, and others can be measured very accurately and may guide heart function assessment and help in diagnosing heart failure and cardiomyopathy. Furthermore, AI can serve as a clinical decision support assistant by integrating the echocardiographic data from a patient with other data – the history of the patient and test results. In this way, treatment planning would be more and more individualized, and then CVDs would better be managed [16].

10.5.2 *Impact of Computer Vision on Radiology*

The automation of image analysis diminishes the task load on radiologists while also increasing diagnosis speed. In an emergency environment, those conditions call for timely interventions to impact good outcomes for the patient. For instance, with computer vision tools, one can quickly identify signs or symptoms of life-threatening conditions such as pulmonary embolism or aortic dissection on a CT scan leading to time-sensitive decisions about treatment. The application of real-time feedback will be very helpful in the efficiency of radiological workflow in terms of allowing healthcare providers to prioritize cases.

Computer vision technologies standardize radiology interpretations apart from increasing the speed and accuracy of diagnoses. This is achieved through reducing variability associated with human interpretation. This turns out to produce consistency in the diagnosis between several radiologists and institutions because of a lack of variability associated with each radiologist's interpretation. It is important especially when one has a large healthcare system where a number of practitioners are interpreting the same imaging study. This has resulted in standardized interpretation that implies more reliable management strategies for patients and minimized chances of misdiagnosis.

Though computer vision brings many benefits to radiology, there are still issues at play. Important ones include data privacy, algorithmic transparency, and the requirement for proper validation that meets the clinical safety and effectiveness standards. Aside from these, even as computer vision significantly helps radiologists, it is vital to note that such tools cannot replace human expertise but instead are designed to enhance it. Integration of computer vision into radiology will occur only if there is significant collaboration between technology developers and healthcare professionals with regard to producing systems that ease practice and enhance clinical workflow [17].

10.6 Cloud Computing and IoT in Healthcare

Cloud computing and the IoT are revolutionizing the healthcare area nowadays, to improve data storage, accessibility, and real-time monitoring of a patient's health. The collection of huge amounts of patient data through wearable health trackers, smart sensors, and connected medical equipment can be integrated with cloud computing platforms. This, on the other hand, brings a tremendous improvement in the integration of cloud technology into some very major implications for decision-making, care for personal needs, and good resource management. Cloud computing can scale and adapt by offering healthcare organizations solutions that are flexible enough to accommodate the changing needs of patients while at the same time still being able to adhere to regulatory requirements regarding data privacy, thereby resulting in better patient results and more efficient healthcare procedures.

10.6.1 Cloud-Based Data Processing

Cloud-based data processing is emerging as a modern means of changing the healthcare scenario with an expansive, efficient, and cost-effective solution for dealing with vast sets of medical data. Following EHRs, real-time monitoring of patients, and medical imaging, healthcare organizations face rigid challenges in storing, processing, and analyzing these data. Cloud computing solves the aforementioned problems with flexible infrastructure that enables healthcare providers to access, share, and analyze data securely over the Internet. One of the main advantages might be scalability in cloud-based data processing. Healthcare organizations with extra scalability will, therefore, always be able to scale up or down their storage and processing according to the volume they need without a large investment in physical infrastructure which is a primary characteristic of traditional architectures. The coordination of its providers can also be facilitated by using cloud-based solutions. It can accommodate hundreds of users logging into and accessing patient information in real-time geo-located from anywhere making connectivity that helps coordinate the care between multidisciplinary teams, for instance, radiologists may exchange real-time imaging reports with primary care physicians for prompt treatments and diagnosis.

With this integration, IoT devices with cloud-based data processing are also enabling the real-time monitoring of patient health. For instance, using wearable devices such as a heart rate monitor or even glucose sensors, continuous health information is received and transmitted to the analysis process on the cloud platforms. From here, healthcare providers can remotely access the data and make timely interventions and personalized care strategies that target the unique needs of patients. This would help in controlling chronic diseases in addition to other ways through: reduction in hospitalization, enhancement of life quality, and elevation of the patient's independence [18].

10.6.2 IoT Enabled Devices

Wearable fitness trackers, more resemble a FitBit, a Garmin, or an Apple watch: tracking physical activity as well as other health metrics such as heart rate and sleep patterns. The data will also frequently sync to a cloud-based platform, making it easier for the user and the healthcare provider to track overall health and fitness trends.

Continuous Glucose Monitors (CGMs): Continuous glucose monitoring devices, such as the Dexcom G6 and FreeStyle Libre, are monitored in real-time, giving the diabetic patient a live idea of their blood sugar levels. They do send this through to a smartphone app, making it easy for the patient to monitor his or her glucose levels. This gives them a better way of monitoring their blood sugar levels and warning them of high or low glucose readings.

Telehealth platforms: These are not in the traditional sense. Telehealth platforms would communicate their respective systems with other devices such as IoTs.

They enable remote consultations. Patients may use other devices, such as a digital thermometer or pulse oximeter, to obtain their health data, and they transmit these to the healthcare providers.

Wearable ECG Monitors: Patients may make their own recordings of heart rhythms by using AliveCor KardiaMobile. Using this technology, devices can already detect atrial fibrillation and other irregularities, which could then be transmitted to healthcare professionals for review.

Smart Beds: The IoT sensors in the beds monitor a patient's movement, vital signs, and pressure levels to prevent bedsores and improve patient care. The beds will promptly alert healthcare providers when a patient needs assistance.

Smart pill dispensers: MedaCube, Hero Smart Dispenser: They can remind the patient and alert them and caregivers of a missed dose [19, 20].

10.7 Future Trends

The future would be filled with the possibility of a gigantic leap of intelligent tools and technologies in propelling real-life diseases brought about through the advancements in AI, ML, NLP, and wearable technologies. The most promising advancement will be in predictive analytics, driven by enormous volumes of data emanating from EHRs, wearables, and mobile applications for the identification of populations at risk, for the prediction of outbreaks of disease, and as a means of preventing threats. Only it will be based on genetic, biomarker, and lifestyle data to make the right treatment for every single patient, and therefore lead to better outcomes because the therapy would be more targeted and effective. Finally, AI in CDSS will simplify and standardize day-to-day healthcare practices since it will provide healthcare professionals with real-time recommendations derived from actual evidence. It should enhance diagnostic acuity and patient treatment. COVID-19 is fast-tracking the use of telehealth and remote monitoring to unprecedented levels so that healthcare providers can monitor patients' health metrics using wearables and mobile applications in real-time, ensuring timely interventions and hospital visits are reduced.

NLP technologies will also advance because chatbots and virtual assistants will engage patients to understand complex medical inquiries with clear information. Patient engagement and access to their health conditions will be much more accessible. With the increased use of digital health records in the future, security, and privacy of health data will become a necessity; however, a blockchain offers promise for decentralized information storage and tamper-proofing that would improve the integrity of patient data and give patients control over their own health data. Robotics and AI will continue to be accelerated in the surgical environment with minimally invasive procedures and lead towards intelligent surgical robots that analyze real-time data during surgeries, assist in providing the best outcomes for patients, and even revolutionize the way surgery is done by letting it be done remotely. Mental health awareness is on the rise, and intelligent tools will slowly begin to hook mental health solutions within general healthcare; it will start with focusing on AI-driven applications and lead the way in assessing, supporting, and even intervening. Moreover, future intelligent tools are to focus on community health by bringing SDOH to the horizon of patient care and thus making it possible for healthcare providers to deal with existing health disparities and to develop targeted interventions that go far beyond a mere consideration of patients' broader contexts. As these smarter tools evolve, regulatory and ethical imperatives will also come into play; regulators will need to catch up to ensure patient safety, patient privacy, and ethical standards are maintained, especially concerning the applications of AI technologies responsibly. There will be a need for guidelines on algorithm transparency and accountability to maintain public trust in the innovations. But overall, the future of intelligent tools and techniques in healthcare is huge, promising to not only improve the detection and management of diseases but also help to keep the patient at the center of the care experience through better collaboration with their healthcare providers and with technology developers in the creative building of a healthcare ecosystem that focuses more on proactive care, personalized treatments, and better health outcomes for all.

References

[1] High, Rob. "The era of cognitive systems: An inside look at IBM Watson and how it works." *IBM Corporation, Redbooks* 1 (2012): 16.

[2] Powles, Julia, and Hal Hodson. "Google DeepMind and healthcare in an age of algorithms." *Health and technology* 7.4 (2017): 351–367.

[3] Stephens, Keri. "Radiology partners, Aidoc partner to accelerate the use of artificial intelligence." *AXIS Imaging News* (2021).

[4] Nadu, Tamil. "Detection of suspicious lesions in mammogram using zebra medical vision algorithm." (2018).

[5] Liang, Zilu, and Mario Alberto Chapa-Martell. "Validation of omron wearable blood pressure monitor HeartGuideTM in free-living environments." *International Conference on Wireless Mobile Communication and Healthcare.* Cham: Springer International Publishing, 2020.

[6] Feehan, Lynne M., et al. "Accuracy of Fitbit devices: systematic review and narrative syntheses of quantitative data." *JMIR mHealth and uHealth* 6.8 (2018): e10527.

[7] Debong, Fredrick, Harald Mayer, and Johanna Kober. "Real-world assessments of mySugr mobile health app." *Diabetes Technology & Therapeutics* 21.S2 (2019): S2–35.

[8] Beatty, Alexis L., et al. "VA FitHeart, a mobile app for cardiac rehabilitation: Usability study." *JMIR Human Factors* 5.1 (2018): e8017.

[9] Apps, Top, and Patient Apps. "AsthmaMD is a well designed free patient app for use in monitoring asthma."

[10] O'Daffer, Alison, et al. "Efficacy and conflicts of interest in randomized controlled trials evaluating headspace and calm apps: systematic review." *JMIR Mental Health* 9.9 (2022): e40924.

[11] Darnell, Doyanne, et al. "Predictors of disengagement and symptom improvement among adults with depression enrolled in talkspace, a technology-mediated psycho-therapy platform: naturalistic observational study." *JMIR Formative Research* 6.6 (2022): e36521.

[12] Azevedo, Daniela, Axel Legay, and Suzanne Kieffer. "User Reception of Babylon Health's Chatbot." VISIGRAPP (2, HUCAPP). 2022.

[13] Wan, Evelyn. ""I'm like a wise little person": Notes on the Metal Performance of Woebot the Mental Health Chatbot." *Theatre Journal* 73.3 (2021): E-21.

[14] Shimizu, Hideyuki, and Keiichi I. Nakayama. "Artificial intelligence in oncology." *Cancer Science* 111.5 (2020): 1452–1460.

[15] Du-Harpur, X., et al. "What is AI? Applications of artificial intelligence to dermatology." *British Journal of Dermatology* 183.3 (2020): 423–430.

[16] Alsharqi, Maryam, et al. "Artificial intelligence and echocardiography." *Echo Research & Practice* 5.4 (2018): R115–R125.

[17] Syed, Ali B., and Adam C. Zoga. "Artificial intelligence in radiology: current technology and future directions." *Seminars in Musculoskeletal Radiology*. 22.05 (2018).

[18] Rajabion, Lila, et al. "Healthcare big data processing mechanisms: The role of cloud computing." *International Journal of Information Management* 49 (2019): 271–289.

[19] Goyal, Sukriti, et al. "IoT enabled technology in secured healthcare: Applications, challenges and future directions." *Cognitive Internet of Medical Things for Smart Healthcare: Services and Applications* (2021): 25–48.

[20] Pradhan, Bikash, Saugat Bhattacharyya, and Kunal Pal. "IoT-based applications in healthcare devices." *Journal of Healthcare Engineering* 2021.1 (2021): 6632599.

Chapter 11

Free Space Detection in Medical Image Analysis for Visually Impaired Using Histogram Equalization and Adaptive Region Growing

Natesh M, Hamsaveni M and Chethana H T

11.1 Introduction

Vision is one of the very important human senses and the eyes play a vital role. Vision plays the most important role in human perception of the surrounding environment [1]. Generally, vision impairment is caused due to several reasons such as blindness by birth or various damages to the brain. People who suffer from blindness or are affected by visual impairment face difficulties in movement apart from many other problems. This condition leads the concerned person to be handicapped and need guidance or assistance for every action [1, 2]. Mobility is one of the main problems encountered by visually impaired persons in their daily lives [3]. In order to help blind people various instruments had been developed for rehabilitation of blindness. Over the decades, these people were using navigational aids such as white cane and guide dogs. Long white cane is a traditional mobility tool used to detect

DOI: 10.1201/9781003617013-11

obstacles in the path of the blind person. On the other hand, guide dogs are assistance dogs, trained to lead the visually impaired around obstacles. Due to the development of modern technology, many different types of navigational aids are now available to assist the blinds. They are commonly known as Electronic Travel Aids. Walking safely and confidently without any human assistance in urban or unknown environments is a difficult task for blind people [2]. But still, the developed instruments are not satisfactory for the rehabilitation of blindness [1].

Many researchers have proposed devices for improving blind people's life quality. Human vision abilities are extraordinary to realize images with the imbibed images in the brain, but these also have some limitations such as being tired, slow and not so accurate because of some disease [1, 4]. These limitations may be rectified by using the principles of computer vision system which definitely improves the blind life quality. Few researchers have proposed outdoor navigation devices for vision-affected persons [1]. The aim of computer vision is to make computers "see" by processing images and/or video. By knowing such things as how images are formed, information about the sensors (cameras) and information about the physical world, it is possible to infer information about the world from an image or set of images [5, 6]. For example, one may wish to know the colour of an apple, the width of a printed circuit trace, the size of an obstacle in front of a robot on Mars, the identity of a person's face in a surveillance system, the motion of an object, the vegetation type of the ground below, or the location of tumour in an MRI scan – automatically, from images. Computer vision studies how such tasks can be done and how they can be done robustly and efficiently. Originally seen as a sub-area of artificial intelligence, computer vision has been an active area of research for almost 40 years. Everyday barcode scanners are used in supermarkets and pattern recognition techniques are used for such purposes as identification, bill recognition and address recognition [7].

The goal of computer vision is to enable computers to see the world. By using a camera as the eye of a computer, studies in computer vision seek to develop better means to capture and extract useful visual information from images and videos and to use such information to automatically interpret the beautiful world surrounding us. Applications range from tasks such as industrial machine vision systems which, say, inspect bottles speeding by on a production line, to research into artificial intelligence and computers or robots that can comprehend the world around them. The computer vision and machine vision fields have significant overlap [5, 8]. Computer vision covers the core technology of automated image analysis which is used in many fields. Machine vision usually refers to a process of combining automated image analysis with other methods and technologies to provide automated inspection and robot guidance in industrial applications. As a scientific discipline, computer vision is concerned with the theory behind artificial systems that extract information from images. The image data can take many forms, such as video sequences, views from multiple cameras, or multi-dimensional data from a medical scanner [9].

As a technological discipline, computer vision seeks to apply its theories and models to the construction of computer vision systems. Examples of applications of computer vision include systems for, Controlling processes (e.g., an industrial robot), Navigation (e.g., by an autonomous vehicle or mobile robot), Detecting events (e.g., for visual surveillance or people counting), Organizing information (e.g., for indexing databases of images and image sequences), Modelling objects or environments (e.g., medical image analysis or topographical modelling) and Interaction (e.g., as the input to a device for computer-human interaction). Sub-domains of computer vision include scene reconstruction, event detection, video tracking, object recognition, learning, indexing, motion estimation and image restoration. In most practical computer vision applications, the computers are pre-programmed to solve a particular task, but methods based on learning are now becoming increasingly common [6, 7].

Image-based floor detection [10] is an application of computer vision and it can be incorporated into the navigation of blind people. Here the navigation is based on finding the free space occupancy. By knowing where the floor is, the blind person can avoid obstacles by navigating within the free space. Detecting the floor, the blind person is also able to acquire information that would be useful in constructing a map of the environment, insofar as the floor detection specifically delineates between the floor and the walls. Moreover, localization using an existing map can be guided by floor detection by matching the location of the detected floor with the location of the floor expected from the map. Additional reasons for floor detection [10] include problems such as computing the size of the room. A significant amount of research has focused on the obstacle avoidance problem. In these techniques, the primary purpose is to detect the free space immediately around the blind person rather than the specific wall-floor boundary. Most of these approaches utilize the ground plane constraint assumption to measure whether the disparity or motion of pixels matches the values that would be expected if the points lie on the ground plane.

In this paper, a technique is designed to aid the blind person using edge detection. The technique aims to give the person information about the free space apart from the obstacles around him in all directions for better mobility. The technique comprises three modules, namely the histogram equalization module, segmentation module and Kalman filtering module. In the histogram equalization module, a canny edge detector is employed to detect edges, and subsequently, histogram equalization is carried out. Subsequently, adaptive region growth is employed in the segmentation module to complete the segmentation process. In the Kalman filtering module, the input image is Kalman filtered and compared with the segmented image to have the free space calculation. The comparison is carried out with the help of the OR operator and the resulting figure gives the free space.

11.2 Literature Review

There has been lots of work related to blind person navigation assistance. Some of the works are briefed here. A. Dhanshri And K. R. Kashwan [1] aimed at finding a viable and simple solution for visually challenged persons at a fractional cost. This paper was an effort to report a comprehensive method to design, characterize and test electronic systems for the aid of blind persons. The simulation tests were carried out using MATLAB and images of test objects were acquired online by using the NI-LabVIEW platform. The main objectives were to acquire an image of an obstacle, identify it, measure a distance from the current location and finally convert text into synthesized. João José et al. [2] designed and presented a SmartVision prototype. It was a small, cheap and easily wearable navigation aid for blind and visually impaired persons. Its functionality addresses global navigation for guiding the user to some destiny, and local navigation for negotiating paths, sidewalks and corridors, with avoidance of static as well as moving obstacles. Local navigation applies to both indoor and outdoor situations. They focused on local navigation: the detection of path borders and obstacles in front of the user and just beyond the reach of the white cane, such that the user can be assisted in centring on the path and alerted to looming hazards. Using a stereo camera worn at chest height, a portable computer in a shoulder-strapped pouch or pocket and only one earphone or small speaker, the system was inconspicuous, it was no hindrance while walking with the cane, and it does not block normal surround sounds. The vision algorithms were optimized such that the system can work at a few frames per second.

Nithya and Shravani [3] presented an electronic travel aid for blind people to navigate safely and quickly, an obstacle detection system using UVC camera-based visual navigation has been considered. The proposed system detected obstacles up to 300 cm via sonar and sends feedback in the form of a beep sound to inform the person about its location. In addition to this, a UVC webcam was connected to 32-bit ARM microcontroller, which supports features and algorithms for designing blind people's guidance sticks. This supported image processing which was used to process images and give voice responses after detection which was used for finding the properties of the obstacle in particular, in the context of the work. Identification of human presence was based on face detection and object detection. The algorithms were implemented in open CV, which runs on the LINUX environment. Lorenzo Picinali et al. [4] investigated the possibilities of assisting blind individuals in learning a spatial environment configuration through listening of audio events and their interactions with these events within a virtual reality experience. A comparison of two types of learning through auditory exploration was performed: *in situ* real displacement and active navigation in a virtual architecture. The virtual navigation rendered only acoustic information. Results for two groups of five participants showed that interactive exploration of virtual acoustic room simulations can provide sufficient information for the construction of coherent spatial mental maps, although some variations were found between the two environments tested in the experiments. Furthermore, the mental representation of the virtually navigated environments preserved topological and metric properties, as was found through actual navigation.

Bhuvanesh Arasu and Senthil Kumaran [11] proposed a device to help a visually challenged person live like any other normal person on this planet without any personal guide. This device made use of the concept of echolocation used by bats. Several components were used in developing this device so called the blind man's eye such as an ultrasonic sound emitter, ultrasonic sound receiver, microcontroller, camera and a steel rod. To sense the size of the object, the intensity of the returned ultrasonic wave was used. Using Doppler's Effect, the object's speed, direction and motion (towards or away) of the object was determined. Making use of angle detection, the technique determined if the person was walking looking down or keeping his head straight. Dijkstra's algorithm was used to find the shortest path in order to direct the blind user from the current path. The Doppler's effect was to find the relative motion of the objects, towards or away from the user. Vincent Gaudissar [12] described an embedded device dedicated to blind or visually impaired people. The main aim of the system was to build an automatic text-reading assistant using existing hardware associated with innovative algorithms. A personal digital assistant (PDA) was chosen because it combined small-size, computational resources and low-cost price. Three key technologies were necessary: text detection, optical character recognition and speech synthesis. Moreover, to be as efficient as possible, a specific interface was created to answer blind people's requests.

Fernandes et al. [13] presented a platform to handle and provide geographic information, including accessibility-oriented features. This geographic information system (GIS) was part of a wider project, called SmartVision. The aim of this project was to create a system that allowed blind users to navigate the University of Trás-os-Montes and Alto Douro campus. The GIS platform, together with other modules of the SmartVision system prototype, provided information to blind users, assisting their navigation and giving alerts of nearby points-of-interest or obstacles. Together with the GIS platform, the paper also described the handling of accessibility information by the SmartVision prototype, namely the Navigation Module, the Computer Vision Module and the Interface Module. Anke M. Brock et al. [14] presented a comparison of the usability of a classical raised-line map versus an interactive map composed of a multitouch screen, a raised-line overlay and audio output. Both maps were tested by 24 blind participants. They measured usability as efficiency, effectiveness and satisfaction. Our results showed that replacing braille with simple audio-tactile interaction significantly improved efficiency and user satisfaction. Effectiveness was not related to the map type but depended on users' characteristics as well as the category of assessed spatial knowledge. Long-term evaluation of acquired spatial information revealed that maps, whether interactive or not, were useful in building robust survey-type mental representations in blind users. These results were encouraging as they show that interactive maps were a good solution for improving map exploration and cognitive mapping in visually impaired people.

Kammoun et al. [15] proposed The NAVIG project which covered important drawback factors: (1) positioning accuracy provided by these devices was not sufficient to guide a VI pedestrian, (2) systems were based on Geographical Information Systems not adapted to pedestrian mobility and (3) the guidance methods should be adapted to the task of pedestrian navigation. The NAVIG project aimed to answer all these limitations through a participatory design framework with the VI and orientation and mobility instructors. The NAVIG device aimed to complement conventional mobility aids (i.e., white cane and guide dog), while also adding unique features to localize specific objects in the environment, restore some visuomotor abilities and assist navigation. Wersényi, György et al. [16] presented a virtual localization for blind persons. In order for blind people to better use personal computers, an auditory virtual environment was used to present information that might otherwise be available only with vision. Auditory objects can be spatially placed in the virtual environment if the user can successfully identify their location. In contrast to sighted subjects, blind subjects were better at detecting movements in the horizontal plane around the head, localizing static frontal audio sources and orientation in a 2-D virtual audio display. On the other hand, sighted subjects performed better in identifying ascending sound sources in the vertical plane and detecting static sources in the back.

11.3 Motivation

Vision plays the most important role in human perception about the surrounding environment and mobility is one of the main problems encountered by visually impaired persons in their daily life. Many researchers have proposed devices for improving blind people's life quality. Many researchers have proposed devices for improving blind people's life quality. Human vision abilities are extraordinary to realize images with the imbibed images in the brain, but these also have some limitations like being tired, slow and not so accurate because of some disease. These limitations may be rectified by using the principles of computer vision system which definitely improves the blind life quality. Image-based floor detection is an application of computer vision and it can be incorporated into the navigation of blind people. Depth estimation in 2-D images is a difficult task and to do this one has to really estimate the depth of individual objects and the magnitude of all the images has to be computed by applying different techniques.

11.4 Free Space Measurement for Blind Person Using Histogram Equalization and Adaptive Region Growing

The proposed technique is designed to aid the blind person by giving the person information about the free space apart from the obstacles around him in all directions for better mobility. The technique employs histogram equalization and adaptive region growth. The technique comprises three modules, namely the histogram equalization module, segmentation module and Kalman filtering module. The block diagram of the proposed technique is given in Figure 11.1.

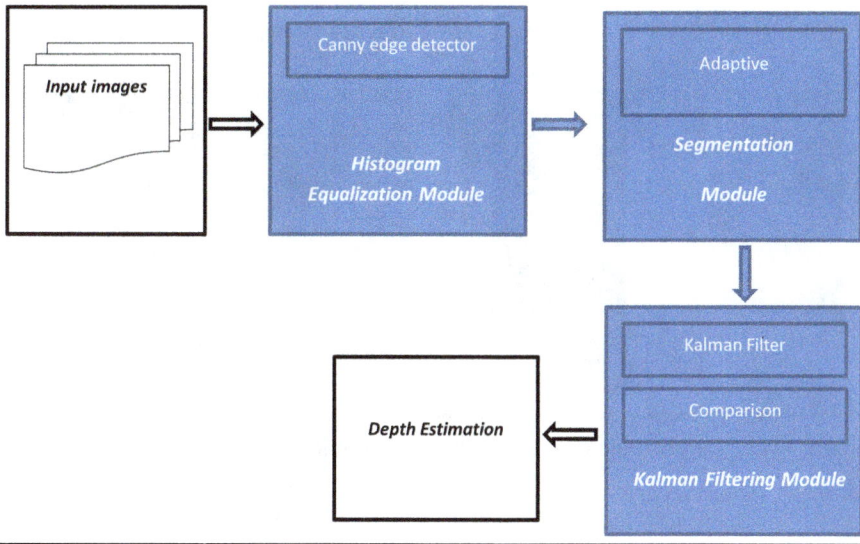

Figure 11.1   Block diagram of the proposed technique.

11.5 Histogram Equalization Module

The first step of the approach detects intensity edges by applying the canny edge detection [17] and then applying histogram equalization. Edges are significant local changes of intensity in an image. Edges typically occur on the boundary between two different regions in an image. Edge detection aims at identifying points in a digital image at which the image brightness changes sharply or, more formally, has discontinuities which are typically organized into a set of curved line segments termed edges. In our technique, we employ a canny edge detector. The Canny edge detector is an edge detection operator that uses a multi-stage algorithm to detect a wide range of edges in images. Canny edge detector has the advantage of having a low error rate.

For canny edge detection, initially, the image is converted to a grey scale image, and the following processes [18] are carried out:

■ Smoothing
■ Finding gradients
■ Non-maximum suppression
■ Double thresholding
■ Edge tracking by hysteresis

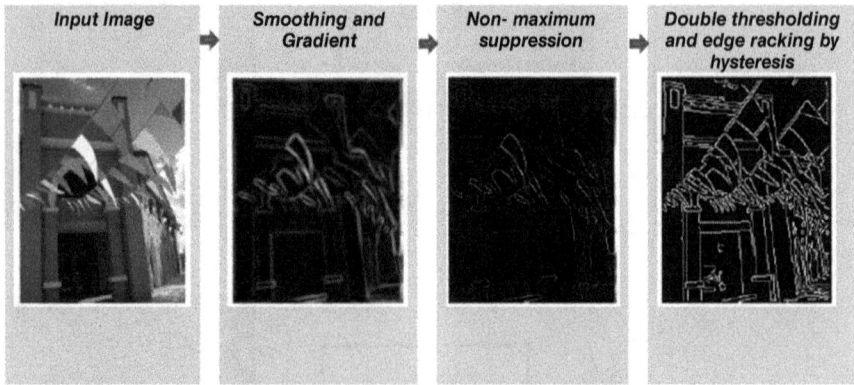

Figure 11.2 Canny edge detection steps for sample image.

The steps involved and its output for a sample image are given in Figure 11.2.

1. Smoothing

   The smoothing process consists of blurring of the image by use of a Gaussian filter to remove noise [19]. It is inevitable that all images taken from a camera will contain some amount of noise. To prevent that noise is mistaken for edges, noise must be reduced. Therefore, the image is first smoothed by applying a Gaussian filter. Let the image in consideration be represented by $I(x, y)$ and $G(x, y)$ be the Gaussian filter, then the resultant smoothened image $S(x, y)$ can be represented by:

$$S(x, y) = G(x, y) \otimes I(x, y) \tag{11.1}$$

2. Gradient

   The objective here is to mark the edges where the gradients of the image have large magnitudes. The Canny algorithm basically finds edges where the grayscale intensity of the image changes the most. These areas are found by determining the gradients of the image. Gradients at each pixel in the smoothed image are determined by applying what is known as the Sobel-operator. The first step is to approximate the gradient in the x- and y-direction respectively by applying the kernels. The gradient magnitudes (R) can then be determined as an Euclidean distance measure by applying the law of Pythagoras given by:

$$|R| = \sqrt{R_X^2 + R_Y^2} \tag{11.2}$$

   where

   R_X and R_Y are the gradients in the x- and y-directions, respectively.

3. Non-maximum suppression

   The purpose of this step is to convert the blurred edges in the image of the gradient magnitudes to sharp edges. Basically, this is done by preserving all local maxima in the gradient image and deleting everything else. Here initially round the gradient direction to nearest 45°. Then, compare the edge strength of the current pixel with the edge strength of the pixel in the positive and negative gradient direction. If the edge strength of the current pixel is the largest; preserve the value of the edge strength. If not, remove the value.

4. Double thresholding

   It is carried out to determine the potential edges which are carried out by thresholding. The edge pixels remaining after the non-maximum suppression step are (still) marked with their strength pixel-by-pixel. Many of these will probably be true edges in the image, but some may be caused by noise or colour variations for instance due to rough surfaces. The simplest way to discern between these would be to use a threshold so that only edges stronger than a certain value would be preserved. The Canny edge detection algorithm uses double thresholding. Edge pixels stronger than the high threshold are marked as strong; edge pixels weaker than the low threshold are suppressed and edge pixels between the two thresholds are marked as weak.

5. Edge tracking by hysteresis

   Here, final edges are determined by suppressing all edges that are not connected to a very strong edge. Strong edges are interpreted as "certain edges", and can immediately be included in the final edge image. Weak edges are included if and only if they are connected to strong edges. The logic is of course that noise and other small variations are unlikely to result in a strong edge. Thus, strong edges would only be due to true edges in the original image. The weak edges can either be due to true edges or noise/colour variations. The latter type will probably be distributed independently of edges on the entire image, and thus, only a small amount will be located adjacent to strong edges. Weak edges due to true edges are much more likely to be connected directly to strong edges.

6. Histogram Equalization

   Histogram equalization is a technique for adjusting image intensities to enhance contrast. This method usually increases the global contrast of many images, especially when the usable data of the image is represented by close contrast values. Through this adjustment, the intensities can be better distributed on the histogram. This allows for areas of lower local contrast to gain a higher contrast. Histogram equalization accomplishes this by effectively spreading out the most frequent intensity values. The method is useful in images with backgrounds and foregrounds that are both bright or dark. A key advantage of the method is that it is a fairly straightforward technique and an invertible operator.

11.6 Segmentation Module

Subsequently, after the edge detection and histogram equalization, the segmentation of the image is carried out using adaptive region growing. Region growing is a simple image segmentation method based on the region [30]. It is also classified as a pixel-based image segmentation method since it involves the selection of initial seed points. This approach to segmentation examines the neighbouring pixels of initial "seed points" and determines whether the pixel neighbours should be added to the region or not based on certain conditions. The process is iterated to yield different regions. In a normal region growing technique, the neighbour pixels are examined by only the "intensity" constraint. For this, a threshold level for intensity value is set and those neighbour pixels that satisfy this threshold are selected for region growth. The normal region growth has the drawback that noise or variation of intensity may result in holes or over-segmentation. Another drawback is that the method may not distinguish the shading of the real images. For improving the normal region growth and effectively tackling the drawbacks of normal region growth, adaptive region growth is proposed. Normally, a segmented area by region growing may consist of small holes. In order to avoid this scenario, the proposed region growing negates small holes inside the regions.

The region growing is a three-step process that consists of gridding, selection of seed point and applying region growing to the point. In gridding, a single image is divided into several smaller images by drawing an imaginary grid over it. That is, gridding results in converting the image into several smaller grid images. The grids are usually square in shape and the grid number to which the original image is split is a variable. Gridding results in smaller grids so that analysis can be carried out easily. The initial step in region growing for the grid formed is to select a seed point for the grid. The initial region begins as the exact location of the seed. Then, histogram analysis is carried out to find out the seed point of the grid. The histogram is found for every pixel in the grid. As the image is a greyscale image, the values of this image are from 0 to 255. For every grid, the histogram value that comes most frequently is selected as the seed point pixel. From this, any one of the seed point pixels is taken as the seed point for the grid.

After finding out the seed point, the region is grown from it. Here the neighbouring pixels are compared with the seed point and if the neighbour pixel satisfies intensity constraints, then the region is grown else it is not grown to that pixel. The intensity threshold defines the maximum value by the neighbour pixel value that can differ from the pixel in consideration. Suppose the pixel has the intensity value I_p, and the neighbouring pixel has the value I_N and the intensity threshold is set as T_I, then if $\| I_p - I_N \| \leq T_I$, *then* intensity constraint is met and satisfied.

When the intensity constraint is satisfied by a neighbouring pixel, then the region is grown to the neighbour pixel and the region grows. For every grid, the region is grown, and based on these regions' features are extracted. After the process, small areas that are left out are checked for and then negated.

11.7 Kalman Filtering Module

The input image is Kalman filtered and compared with the segmented image to have the free space calculation. The comparison is carried out with the help of the OR operator and the resulting figure gives the free space. Kalman filtering [20] is an algorithm that uses a series of measurements observed over time, containing noise and other inaccuracies, and produces estimates of unknown variables that tend to be more precise than those based on a single measurement alone. The Kalman filter is a recursive estimator. This means that only the estimated state from the previous time step and the current measurement are needed to compute the estimate for the current state. The Kalman filtering algorithm works in a two-step process. In the prediction step, the Kalman filter produces estimates of the current state variables, along with their uncertainties. Once the outcome of the next measurement (necessarily corrupted with some amount of error, including random noise) is observed, these estimates are updated using a weighted average, with more weight being given to estimates with higher certainty.

The Kalman filter model [20] for the system and a particular time instant τ_i is given as shown below:

$$Y_i = n_i Y_i + Z_i \tag{11.3}$$

where Y_i is the n-dimensional vector, n_i is the n x n matrix and Z_i is the random sequence vector in the system. Consider that at time τ_i, there is an n-dimensional vector available which is corrupted by a noise, and then the expression is given as shown below:

$$K_i = R_i Y_i + N_i \tag{11.4}$$

where R_i is called the m x n observation matrix and the vector N_i is the additive noise in the processing. Assuming that the vectors, Z_i and N_i are mutually correlated to one another, which results in the expression:

$$G\left[Z_i N_i^j\right] = \phi; i = 0,1,..... \tag{11.5}$$

where ϕ represents the null matrix. Based on these considerations we derive the equation for the Kalman filtering which is given in the below expression,

$$Y_i = n_i Y_{i-1} + H_i\left[K_i - R_i Y_{i-1}\right] \tag{11.6}$$

Let the input image be represented by I and let the image after the Kalman filtering be represented by K. Let the image after the segmentation be represented by V. Here, the segmented image V is compared with the Kalman-filtered image K, as shown in Figure 11.3.

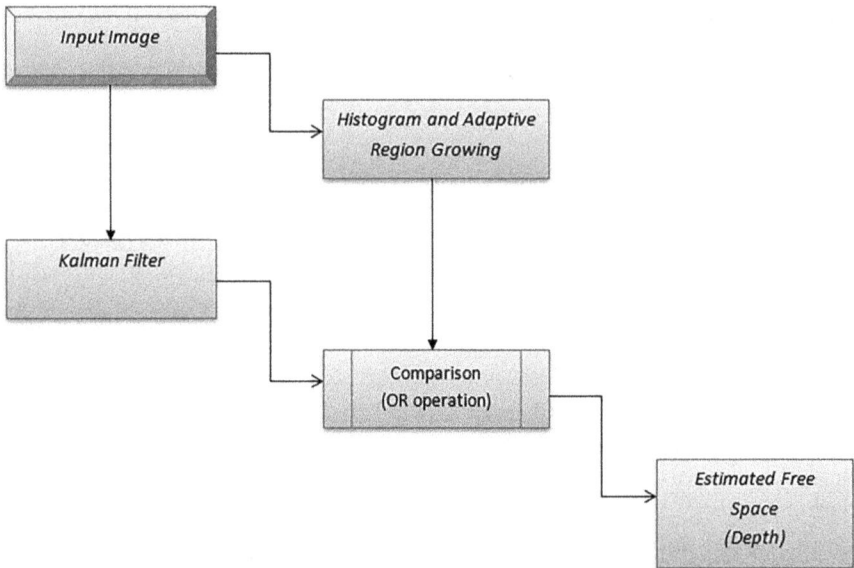

Figure 11.3   Kalman filtering module.

The comparison is carried out using the OR operator. The OR operator typically takes two images as input and outputs a third image whose pixel values are just those of the first mage, ORed with the corresponding pixels from the second. In our case, the Kalman-filtered image is ORed with the segmented image to have the ORed image. The operation is performed straightforwardly in a single pass. It is important that all the input pixel values being operated on have the same number of bits in them or unexpected things may happen. Where the pixel values in the input images are not simple 1-bit numbers, the OR operation is normally carried out individually on each corresponding bit in the pixel values, in a bitwise fashion. The ORed image gives the free space estimation.

11.8 Results and Discussions

The proposed free space measurement technique is analysed with the help of experimental results in this section. In Section 11.8.1, the experimental setup and the evaluation metrics employed are discussed. The simulation results obtained are given in Section 11.8.2 and performance analysis is made in Section 11.8.3.

11.8.1 Experimental Setup and Evaluation Metrics

The proposed technique is implemented using MATLAB on a system having the configuration of 6 GB RAM and 2.8 GHz Intel i-7 processor. The evaluation

Table 11.1 Table Defining the Terms TP, FP, FN, TN

Experimental Outcome	Condition as determined by the Standard of Truth	Definition
Positive	Positive	**True Positive (TP)**
Positive	Negative	**False Positive (FP)**
Negative	Positive	**False Negative (FN)**
Negative	Negative	**True Negative (TN)**

metrics used to evaluate the proposed technique consist of sensitivity, specificity and accuracy. In order to find these metrics, we first compute some of the terms of True positive (TP), True negative (TN), False negative (FN) and False positive (FP) based on the definitions given in Table 11.1.

The evaluation metrics of sensitivity, specificity and accuracy can be expressed in terms of TP, FP, FN and TN. Sensitivity is the proportion of TPs that are correctly identified by a diagnostic test. It shows how good the test is at detecting a disease.

$$\text{Sensitivity} = TP / (TP + FN)$$

Specificity is the proportion of the TNs correctly identified by a diagnostic test. It suggests how good the test is at identifying normal (negative) conditions.

$$\text{Specificity} = TN / (TN + FP)$$

Accuracy is the proportion of true results, either TP or TN, in a population. It measures the degree of veracity of a diagnostic test on a condition.

$$\text{Accuracy} = (TN + TP) / (TN + TP + FN + FP)$$

11.8.2 Simulation Results

In this section, the simulation results obtained for the proposed technique are given. Figure 11.4 gives the simulation results of the input image, floor-marked input image, edge-marked input image, edge detected using canny edge detector, clustered image using FCM, Kalman filtered image, clustered image and output image. In the output image, free space is marked in red.

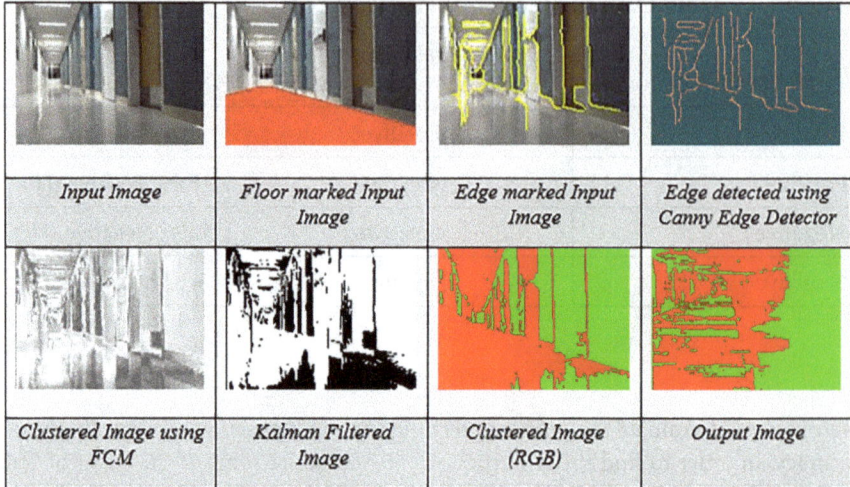

Input Image	Floor marked Input Image	Edge marked Input Image	Edge detected using Canny Edge Detector
Clustered Image using FCM	Kalman Filtered Image	Clustered Image (RGB)	Output Image

Figure 11.4 Simulation results.

11.8.3 Performance Analysis

In this section, the performance of the proposed technique is analysed with the use of evaluation metrics of sensitivity, specificity and accuracy.

Inferences from Figures 11.5 and 11.6 and Table 11.2:

■ Figures 11.5, 11.6 and Table 11.2 give the evaluation metrics obtained for the proposed technique.
■ The evaluation in consideration includes TP, FP, TN, FN, sensitivity, specificity and accuracy.
■ Figure 11.5 and Table 11.1 give the evaluation metrics obtained by varying the cluster size. Cluster sizes in consideration are 2, 3 and 4.
■ From the results, it can be seen that all cases have yielded good results. Amongst, the best results came when cluster size was taken for 2.
■ The highest sensitivity, specificity and accuracy came at about 0.90, 0.50 and 0.71, respectively (when cluster size was taken as 2).
■ Figure 11.6 gives the average obtained considering all cluster sizes.
■ The average TP, TN, FP and FN came about 0.79, 0.5, 0.5 and 0.20, respectively. The average sensitivity, specificity and accuracy came to about 0.79, 0.50 and 0.67, respectively.
■ The high average values indicate the good performance of the proposed technique in the area.

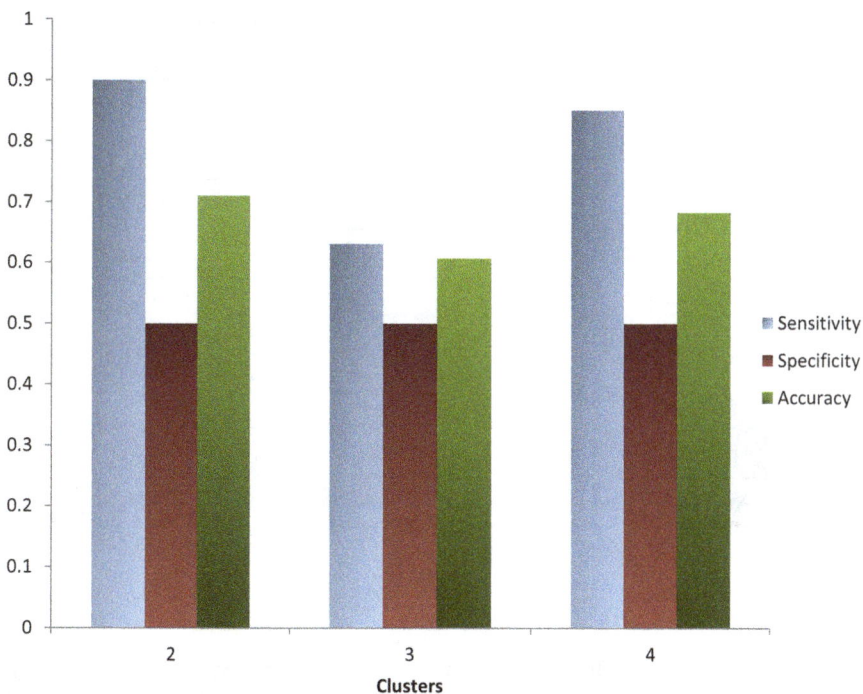

Figure 11.5 Chart of evaluation metric values obtained for varying cluster sizes.

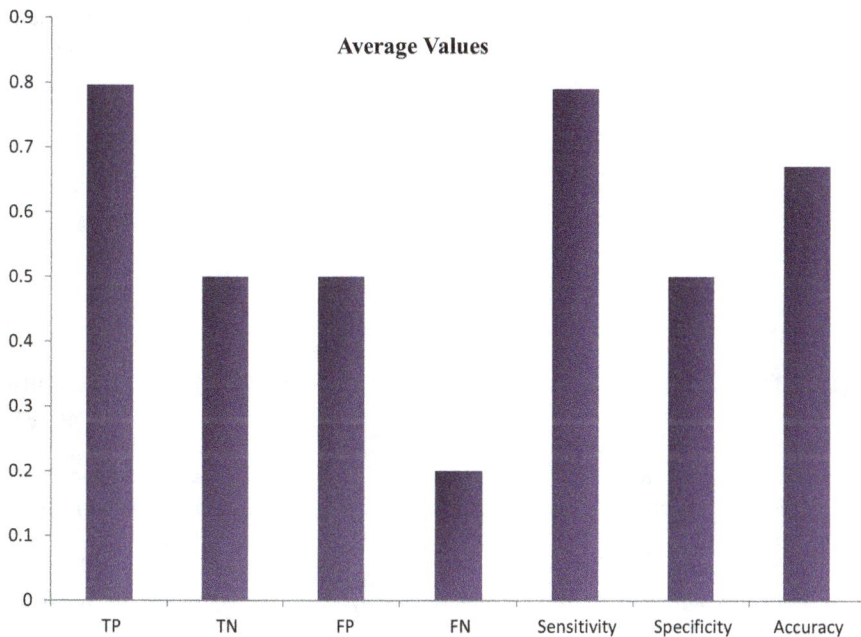

Figure 11.6 Chart of average evaluation metric values obtained.

Table 11.2 Evaluation Metric Values Obtained for Varying Cluster Sizes

	Clusters		
	2	3	4
True Positive	0.90	0.63	0.85
True Negative	0.50	0.50	0.50
False Positive	0.50	0.50	0.50
False Negative	0.10	0.37	0.15
Sensitivity	0.90	0.63	0.85
Specificity	0.50	0.50	0.50
Accuracy	0.71	0.61	0.68

11.9 Conclusion

Free space measurement for blind persons using histogram equalization and adaptive region growth is proposed in this paper. The technique comprises three modules, namely the histogram equalization module, segmentation module and Kalman filtering module. The proposed technique is evaluated under standard evaluation metrics of TP, FP, TN, FN, sensitivity, specificity and accuracy for varying cluster sizes of 2, 3 and 4. The simulation results obtained are plotted. The highest sensitivity, specificity and accuracy came about 0.90, 0.50 and 0.71 and similarly, the average TP, TN, FP and FN came about 0.79, 0.5, 0.5 and 0.20, respectively. Analysing the cluster performance, a cluster size of 2 gave the best results. The high evaluation metric values of sensitivity, specificity and accuracy indicate the good performance of the proposed technique in the area.

References

[1] A. Dhanshri, K. R. Kashwan, "Identification Of Dynamic Objects Using Matlab And Labview For Aiding Blind Person", *International Conference on Electronics and Communication Engineering*, pp. 142–149, 2013.

[2] J. José, M. Farrajota, J. M. Rodrigues and J. H. du Buf, "The smart vision local navigation aid for blind and visually impaired persons", *International Journal of Digital Content Technology and its Applications*, Vol. 5 No. 5, pp. 362–374, 2011.

[3] S. Nithya and A. S. L. Shravani, "Electronic Eye for Visually Impaired Persons", *International Journal of Emerging Technology and Advanced Engineering*, Vol. 3, No. 10, pp. 700–704, 2013.

[4] Lorenzo Picinali, Amandine Afonso, Michel Denis and Brian F.G. Katz, "Exploration of architectural spaces by blind people using auditory virtual reality for the construction of spatial knowledge", *International Journal of Human-Computer Studies*, Vol. 72, No. 4, pp. 393–407, 2014.

[5] O. D. Faugeras. *Three – Dimensional Computer Vision: a Geometric Viewpoint*. MIT Press, 1993.

[6] O. D. Faugeras, "Stratification of three-dimensional vision: Projective, affine, and metric representation," *Journal of the Optical Society of America*, A12:465–484, 1995.

[7] E. H. Elsayed, T. Ahmed Monumentally, A. Farag, The CardEye: A Trinocular Active Vision System, Springer Berlin/Heidelberg, Vol 2095/2001.

[8] Z. Zhang, "Flexible Camera Calibration by Viewing a Plane from Unknown Orientation," ICCV '97, 1997.

[9] N. Avinash, S. Murali, "Camera Center Estimation Using Vanishing Points", *IEEE 1st International Conference on Signal and Image Processing*, 2006, Volume 1, 467.

[10] Yinxiao Li and Stanley T. Birchfield, "Image-based segmentation of indoor corridor floors for a mobile robot", *IEEE International Conference on Intelligent Robots and Systems (IROS)*, pp. 837–843, 2010.

[11] Bhuvanesh Arasu and Senthil Kumaran, "Blind Man's Artificial EYE An Innovative Idea to Help the Blind", *International Journal of Engineering Development and Research*, pp. 205–208, 2014.

[12] Vincent Gaudissart, Silvio Ferreira, Céline Thillou, Bernard Gosselin, "Mobile Reading Assistant for Blind People", *Conference Speech and Computer*, pp. 538–544, 2004.

[13] H. Fernandes, N. Conceição, H. Paredes, A. Pereira, P. Araújo and J. Barroso, "Providing accessibility to blind people using GIS", *Universal Access in the Information Society*, Vol. 11, No. 4, pp 399–407, 2012.

[14] Anke M. Brocka, Philippe Truilleta, Bernard Oriolaa, Delphine Picardb and Christophe Jouffraisa, "Interactivity improves usability of geographic maps for visually impaired people", *Human–Computer Interaction*, Vol. 30, No. 2, pp. 156–194, 2015.

[15] S. Kammouna, G. Parseihianc, O. Gutierreza, A. Brilhaulta, A. Serpaa, M. Raynala, B. Oriolaa, M.J.-M. Macéa, M. Auvrayc, M. Denisc, S.J. Thorpeb, P. Truilleta, B.F.G. Katzc and C. Jouffraisa, "Navigation and space perception assistance for the visually impaired: The NAVIG project", *IRBM*, Vol. 33, No. 2, pp. 182–189, 2012.

[16] Wersényi György, "Virtual localization by blind persons", *JAES* Vol. 60, No. 7/8, pp. 568–579, 2012.

[17] Azernikov Sergei. Sweeping solids on manifolds. In *Symposium on Solid and Physical Modeling*, 249–255, 2008.

[18] F. Mai, Y. Hung, H. Zhong, and W. Sze. A hierarchical approach for fast and robust ellipse extraction. *Pattern Recognition*, 41(8):2512–2524, August 2008.

[19] W. K. Pratt, *Digital Image Processing*, 4th Edition, John Wiley & Sons, Inc., Los Altos, CA, 2007.

[20] S. J. Julier and J. K. Uhlmann, "Unscented filtering and nonlinear estimation," *Proc. IEEE*, vol. 92, no. 3, pp. 401–422, 2004.

Index

Pages in *italics* refer to figures and pages in **bold** refer to tables.